A Prescription for 2008

A Prescription for 2008

◆

What the Next President Needs to Know About Health Reform

Sven Robert Larson

iUniverse, Inc.

New York Lincoln Shanghai

A Prescription for 2008
What the Next President Needs to Know About Health Reform

iUniverse books may be ordered through booksellers or by contacting:

iUniverse
2021 Pine Lake Road, Suite 100
Lincoln, NE 68512
www.iuniverse.com
1-800-Authors (1-800-288-4677)

The views expressed in this work are solely those of the author and do not necessarily reflect the views of the publisher, and the publisher hereby disclaims any responsibility for them.

ISBN-13: 978-0-595-43732-0 (pbk)
ISBN-13: 978-0-595-88063-8 (ebk)
ISBN-10: 0-595-43732-X (pbk)
ISBN-10: 0-595-88063-0 (ebk)

Printed in the United States of America

To my son, Ivan

Contents

THE MOST EXCITING ELECTION IN A LONG TIME!

The 2008 election will not be a national security election. The next president will not be a national security president. While national security will still be an important part of the president's agenda, domestic issues will rise to the top.

Health reform will be the most important among them. It will be so important, in fact, that the 44th president of the United States probably will go down in history as a health reform president.

Early candidates are picking up on this. The "big name" Democrats, Barack Obama, John Edwards and Hillary Clinton, have all expressed support for Canadian-style universal, single-payer health care. Clinton has the strongest track record in pursuing universal health care, but Edwards and Obama have made it very clear that they share the same views.

What Obama, Edwards and Clinton have in health policy, they lack in leadership skills. It is almost exactly the other way around with Mayor Rudolph Giuliani, commonly viewed as an early Republican frontrunner. He has excellent leadership and crisis management skills. He also has an asset that will come in very handy in Washington: he has a proven track record of dealing with hardheaded liberals (there are lots of them in New York City …).

At the same time, he does not have a health policy worth mentioning. This is too bad, because health policy is going to be the biggest domestic issue in 2008.

Fortunately, America's Mayor does not have to look far for advice. A fellow Republican presidential hopeful, Governor Mitt Romney, has the strongest health reform credentials of any likely 2008 candidate, Democrat or Republican. His market-based reform in Massachusetts has great potentials at the national level and is a strong contender in a run-off against a Clinton-style universal health alternative.

It will be a dream race in 2008—yes!—if both candidates have strong, active health policies in their platforms. That way voters will have a genuine chance to compare two distinctly different, carefully designed and well argued alternatives.

Only good can come out of that. Many people say that differences divide us, but that is the case only when differences become personal. So long as we keep the differences to the issues, they enlighten us. Furthermore, health care reform is directly relevant to all of us. Just like food, shelter and energy, we depend on it to have a good daily life. Just as we see the difference between good and bad food, we see the difference between good and bad health care.

What must not happen is that the Republicans fail to develop a good health reform plan. That way they would lose the White House, and America would lose its health care freedom. Whoever the Democratic nominee will be in 2008, he or she will definitely push for universal, single payer health care run by the federal government (and paid for by $2,000,000,000,000 worth of health care taxes).

But even if a Republican wins the White House in '08 without pushing for health reform, he should not just kick back and think that he does not have to do anything. Many states are probing universal, single payer health care on their own. From Maine to California, state legislatures have voted on, or will soon vote on, single payer systems. If the federal government does nothing to promote free-market based health reform there is a great risk that we will get universal, single payer health care through the state back door, so to speak.

With that in mind, I am discussing two probable alternatives for health reform in the 2008 election campaign. I discuss a "Hillary Care II" plan that, without copycatting, builds on the 1994 Clinton plan. It is the most likely Democratic proposal. I also discuss a Romney plan as a base for a Republican alternative. While the Romney model has many positive elements, it needs some important changes before it can be a credible contender in '08.

To make the reasoning a bit simpler, I refer to Senator Clinton and Governor Romney as the two front runners for 2008. That does not mean that I expect—or even want—them to be the front runners. We could very well end up with Senator Obama vs. Mayor Giuliani, or John Edwards vs. Mitt Romney, or …

Seen strictly from the health policy perspective, a Clinton-Romney contest would be ideal. Therefore, let us pretend that they will be the front runners.

A health-care dominated election would not only benefit America, but it would also be good for the two major parties. They would get a chance to re-focus their agendas and "get back to basics" ideologically. Health reform is one of the purest ideological issues in domestic policy. It puts individual freedom and small government against redistribution and big government in a way that few other issues do. This makes it a complex issue, but it also makes it important, almost indispensable, to both parties. Health reform will encourage internal and public discussions on what it really means to be a socialist, a liberal, a conservative or a libertarian.

In fact, focus on health policy might actually help the Democrats become constructive and visionary on the domestic arena just as some Republicans have. Mitt Romney is a good example. His health reform in Massachusetts provides the Republicans with a clear, actionable health reform plan that is based in traditional conservative principles such as individual freedom and responsibility; free markets and free enterprise; and social responsibility. The Romney model is appealing to Republican voters, including conservatives who abandoned the Republican party in 2006.

The Massachusetts reform might not be perfect, but it was the brainchild of a governor who had to work with one of the nation's most left leaning state legislatures. That gives Mitt Romney a lot of credit in working for national health reform.

His input into the debate is needed. If Democrats are unchallenged in the health care debate, they will most likely win the election and go ahead with a universal, single payer model. Such a reform would let the federal government take over our entire health system. It would constitute an unprecedented expansion of the federal government. For the fiscal year of 2008, the federal government's budget will be about $2.9 trillion. With a universal, single payer system, it would grow by 55 percent literally over night. The federal government would take over not only private spending ($1 trillion) but also state level health expenditures ($400 billion). Together with the federal government's existing health spending, a federal health care agency, running a national single payer system, would have a budget of $2 trillion per year.

The federal government would be one third of our entire economy. Then we add the states, counties, cities …

A Romney-style reform would take us in the opposite direction. It would create a national market for private health insurance, combined with Medicaid for low income families. The government would regulate, but not take over, one of the biggest markets in the country. By stopping short of socializing the health system, the Romney model emphasizes private responsibility and opportunity.

These differences between a Clinton-style reform and a Romney model are not just theoretical. They are much more than that. Europe and Canada have had many troubling, very tangible experiences with their universal health systems. Waiting lists and health rationing have become serious problems. Backers of such ideas here in America have thus far failed to explain how they are going to copy European or Canadian models without also copying their downsides.

In the midst of all the criticism of universal health care, we should also acknowledge that the proponents of such ideas are right in one important respect: our current health system is not working well. Some 45 million Americans are uninsured—some for only a short time, others for years. Even though many of them make enough money to be able to afford health insurance, the majority have no such choice because premiums are too high. Onerous government regulations, and monopolization of the health insurance market, are among the culprits behind the cost problem.

While it is right to criticize universal health insurance, it is incumbent upon those who do, to offer an alternative, a market-based solution that is more than just a facelift.

Governor Romney has done this. Is his model the free market answer? Not yet. But with a few reforms, he might actually hit the nail right on. And if Governor Romney does not win the Republican nomination in 2008, he will have something to teach whoever does win the nomination.

You cannot go up against Senator Clinton—or even Senator Obama—without a credible health reform plan. Health Savings Accounts and tax breaks for health insurance purchases are good reforms but severely insufficient.

Therefore, the Romney plan is almost like a God sent opportunity for the Republicans. They have been fumbling around for a long time to unite around a good alternative to Hillary Care II.

This is their chance.

Once again—let me stress that inaction is not an option. Health reform is coming even if our next president does nothing about it. More than a dozen states are pursuing or considering their own health care reform bills. Most of the state-level reform proposals are about single payer systems. Most of those bills have not led to any legislation, but the push for single payer systems at the state level is getting stronger, not weaker. More states are joining in and new bills are constantly introduced.

In other words: if our next president is a Republican who wants to strengthen the free economy, and if that president does nothing to reform our health care system, some of us may end up with single payer health care anyway. Therefore, the stronger a national alternative the Republicans can present in 2008, the better it will be for our health care.

WHY THE ROMNEY MODEL COULD BE A WINNER

Mitt Romney was elected governor of Massachusetts in 2002. Prior to that he had executive experience from the private sector, both at the helm of Bain Capital—a venture capital firm—and the 2002 Winter Olympics in Salt Lake City. During his years as governor he profiled himself as a fiscal conservative and tried to streamline government operations. It is fair to say that before his health care reform, he was a good but not remarkable governor.

What made his gubernatorial years unique was his health insurance reform, signed into law in April 2006. This is the first comprehensive effort by an influential Republican to come up with a workable answer to the calls for socialized health care. The model is not perfect as it is, but it is a big step forward. If Governor Romney is ever elected president, his model for health reform could elevate him to the highest ranks among our presidents.

So what is his model all about? Here is a brief summary:

- Every resident of Massachusetts must have health insurance. If you do not have it by a certain date, the state will fine you.

- The state creates a health insurance Connector through which private citizens can shop for an insurance that meets their needs and their budget.

- Every plan sold through the Connector must meet each and everyone of the state's 40 coverage mandates. A coverage mandate is a health benefit (contraceptives, hair prostheses, in vitro fertilization, substance abuse treatment) that an insurance plan must provide.

- The state will pay all of, or subsidize, insurance premiums for people who make up to 300 percent of the Federal Poverty Limit.

- The state "expects" insurance plans to cost about $200 per month (today, the national average is $833 per month for a family plan).

Overall, this is not a full fledged private, market based reform, as Governor Romney presents it on his website.[1] It comes with some heavy handed government regulations, especially the state coverage mandates. That said, though, there are some intriguing upsides to the model that Governor Romney deserves a lot of credit for.

The upsides

The most important upside is actually something that is *not* in the Romney model: socialization of all health care. Unlike a universal, single payer system, the Romney model does not give the government a health insurance monopoly. Furthermore, it does not turn physicians and nurses into state employees (which is what happens in a Scandinavian-style socialized health system). Better still, the Romney model does not turn clinics and hospitals into state property.

Bottom line: it does not burden taxpayers with every single dime of people's health care costs.

Granted, the model will cost taxpayers some $5 billion, five times more than what the state of Massachusetts itself has estimated that the reform would cost.[2] But this is still a far cry from the $40+ billion that Massachusetts taxpayers would have to cough up if the state instead had opted for a universal, single payer system.

Instead of putting the government at the center, the model has a Connector, effectively a health insurance market place. It encourages consumers to educate themselves on insurance plans and it makes it easier to compare plans and premiums. Insurance providers will have to compete for business and thereby be forced to improve their offers—just as they should on a free market.

The model's third upside is that everybody will be covered. It not only comes with a mandate that says "you get insurance or ...", but it also has an in-built guarantee that if you cannot afford insurance, the government will provide it for you at the expense of taxpayers.

This list of upsides may not be long as a weekend shopping list, but these three distinctly positive features actually make this model unique. They also give it great potential for the future. In particular, they make the model an intriguing candidate for national reform. Since the Romney model will not go into effect in Massachusetts until July 1, 2007, we cannot know at this point how well it will actually work. There is a real possibility that the downsides will be too heavy a burden for the model, but even if that were to happen, they are manageable and can easily be addressed by the state legislature.

The downsides

The single biggest downside to the plan is that it dictates what health benefits every insurance plan must cover. Massachusetts has 40 such mandates, which means that insurance buyers pre-pay for a whole range of benefits that they will probably never use.

Some of the mandates that health plans have to cover in Massachusetts are: breast reconstruction, chiropractors, contraceptives, hair prostheses, in vitro fertilization, dentists, optometrists, podiatrists and social worker services.

Each of these mandates add to the premium that a health insurance buyer has to pay each month. As an example, just the in vitro fertilization mandate can be responsible for as much as $40 per month on an $800 policy. And you have to pay for it, even if you will never use the service.

It sounds like a good idea to buy coverage for a lot of things "just in case", but the end result is that health insurance becomes a lot more costly. In fact, research shows[3] that states with many mandates have more uninsured residents than states with few mandates.

If the Romney model had removed the state coverage mandates, it would have allowed insurance providers to offer, literally, hundreds of different plans through the Connector. Competition and consumer choice would have forcefully kept the cost of insurance down and allowed consumers to get the most bang for their buck.

Another downside to the Romney model is that the state promises to pay for health insurance for anyone who cannot afford it. Technically, the state has to make this promise since it also forces every resident to buy health insurance. But *precisely because* of that mandate, there is a great risk that the state will have to pay for the health insurance of much more people than they expect.

Look at it this way. You are a hard-working entrepreneur with your own little business. You make a reasonable amount of money but due to the nature of your business your stream of income varies from month to month. Your bills, on the other hand, are pretty stable, especially your mortgage and your car payment. Some months you have no margins at all for more expenses, and you are definitely not going to take on another steady bill, because if you do you may end up in the red or your checks will bounce. So you cannot take on the cost of health insurance, at least not for another year.

Your government—the state of Massachusetts—passes a law that says you have to have health insurance. The state is not going to let you wait until you feel that it is prudent to take on another bill. It threatens to fine you unless you buy a plan right away.

What do you do? On the one hand, you do not qualify for free or subsidized health insurance from the state, because you make slightly more than the income caps that the state has put up. On the other hand, you do not want to be fined and listed somewhere as a health insurance delinquent (and God knows what else …).

So your only logical option is to take the state to court. The state forces you to buy something that you cannot afford—hence, they should give it to you for free or subsidize you so you can buy it on your own.

How does the state respond? Let's say they accept the challenge and the case goes to trial. Suppose they win. The court rules that you have to go to the insurance Connector and buy an insurance plan. You can't do that without risking your good financial standing with your bank. But you certainly cannot risk being listed as a criminal (or whatever they will do to you now that you have a court ruling against you). So you bite the bullet, hope for the best and go buy the cheapest plan you can possibly find.

The state has now put an honest, hard working citizen on the brink of financial hardship and made you look like a criminal—only because you do not make enough money to pay another bill.

But suppose instead that you win the case. This is definitely good for you, but the state has now created a precedent that others can use against it. The state will now have to pay for your health insurance, as well as for the insurance of hundreds of thousands of others who cannot take on another bill. This opens big, big floodgates for tax paid health insurance, something that the Romney model has not properly considered.

It is quite possible that the state can see this coming. It is also possible that they will see that if they try to force you to buy health insurance and put yourself in financial jeopardy, they will look like a big bullying bureaucracy that does not care about the little guy. So they may very well choose to avoid a trial. Instead they will be lenient and let a lot of people in on the tax subsidized plans, even though they technically do not qualify.

End result: taxpayers have to dole out a lot more money than they have been told.

Massachusetts is trying to avoid—or, rather, evade—this problem by "expecting" that health plans will not cost more than $200 per month.[4] This "expectation" is written as a subtle threat that if health plans offered through the Connector are not cheap enough, the state may introduce price control.

This means that the state knows that current insurance plans are too expensive for a lot of people. It would be more honest if they admitted that. As it is now, the "expected" $200 per month premium is way, way below the standard cost for health insurance, which is 833 per month.[5]

In fact, *boston.com* reports[6] that precisely this problem is emerging already, in January 2007—months before the Romney plan goes into effect. Hundreds of thousands of Massachusetts residents are claiming that they will not be able to afford insurance even at the subsidized rates that the state provides. The state is being asked to put off the penalty part of the entire plan and give people at least another year to find an affordable health plan.

The state, in turn, is trying to increase the subsidies and cut the share that people pay. This means, of course, higher costs for taxpayers in the other end, as they have to pick up the rest of the tab.

According to the *boston.com* article, there is also concern in the business community that there will not be enough affordable health plans around—in other words, that premiums are not going to come down to the level that the state has determined is affordable.

If that does not happen at all—then what? Will the state intervene with price control? Or will they dramatically expand tax subsidized health care and let taxpayers pay for it, hoping that voters will forgive them on election day?

Promising, despite the downsides

Let me once again stress the problems that the coverage mandates cause. Suppose that the government dictates that every week you have to pre-pay for a certain set of groceries. As you enter the grocery store on Monday, you pay an entrance fee of $400. This pays for a certain combination of produce, bread, dairy, poultry, beef, Kosher products, hygiene products, candy, chips, beer … In return for your $400 you get a weekly voucher that can be used at any grocery store in the state.

But what if you cannot afford to spend $400 per week on groceries? Well, if your income is low enough you can of course apply for food stamps. If you make too much for food stamps, but too little to let you spend some $1,600 per month on groceries, then you will have to go hungry.

Absurd? Of course it is. But this is how coverage mandates work. It shows quite well what problems they create for us when we want to buy health insurance.

At the same time, this is a problem that can be solved rather easily, especially in a national version of the Romney model. If the federal government set up its own health insurance Connector, it would make all health insurance plans in the country available to any buyer, in any state.

The beauty with this is that every state in the country has its own unique set of coverage mandates. Some states impose less than 20 mandates, while some—like Massachusetts—have more than 40. Obviously, a plan with 20 mandates, sold nationwide, would be cheaper than a plan with 40 mandates.

All that is needed is that a plan is registered in one state. (This requirement would protect consumers against fly-by-night insurance providers.) Once a plan has been approved in one state, it can be sold through the federal Connector to any resident of any state, anywhere in the country.

A national Connector is a nice solution for individuals who cannot afford to buy insurance on their own today. But it is also good for employers who want to offer good health benefits to their employees. Big employers who operate in many states can get a so called ERISA exemption from the state coverage mandates, and offer the same plan across the country. Small businesses cannot do that. They are confined to state regulations which, of course, puts them at a disadvantage compared to big corporations as well as competitors in other states.

With a national Connector, small businesses can escape this problem and get better benefits for less money.

We are in dire need of this type of reform. It is a well known fact that a smaller and smaller percentage of working age Americans have private health insurance—including employer's insurance. In the mid-'80s it was four out of five; today it is only two thirds.

There is yet more evidence that we need market-based health reform now. The share of working age Americans who are uninsured has in two decades increased from 15 percent to more than 20 percent.

More regulations, higher costs. Higher costs, fewer are insured.

By creating a national health insurance market through a Romney-style Connector we may actually solve the problem of unaffordable insurance for a long time to come.[7]

Regulations and costs in the Romney model

One big problem with all health reforms is cost containment. The problem does not come from rising costs per se, but from the belief that we can—and should—impose artificial restrictions on health costs. Moreover, there is a widespread belief that we can combine cost containment with today's excellent health care.

It is with health care just like with any other complex product we buy. If we want a high quality builder to build us a high quality house, it is not going to be cheap. If we want to sue someone for something really bad they did to us, we do not want some $25-an-hour attorney who cannot tell Habeas Corpus from Corpus Christi.

Sure—health insurance companies take their fair share, and perhaps a bit more, out of what we pay for our insurance. And pharmaceutical companies make sure that their bottom line is not exactly razor thin either. But those profits are not the main drive behind the cost of health insurance. For one, pharmaceutical companies take tremendous risks when they start developing new medicines. If they cannot look forward to a good profit, then why bother?

We do not bring down the cost of health insurance by somehow regulating away the profits of insurance companies and the pharmaceutical industry.

We do it by promoting competition and consumer choice.

Unfortunately, the Romney model suffers from a slight case of cost containment delusion. It assumes that there will be a lot of dirt cheap health insurance offerings through the Connector, and that the entire reform will only cost taxpayers $1 billion.

This is a dicey assumption. There is no analysis behind the Romney model to back up its cost containment assumption. In fact, we can easily show that taxpayers may end up footing a bill of $4–5 billion for the Romney plan.

We discussed part of the problem before, when we imagined an entrepreneur who takes the state to court because he cannot afford insurance, even though the state (implicitly) assumes that he can.

Here is another part of the cost containment problem. People who do not have health insurance, despite the mandate, can still get health care at no cost to them. The state will pay for their care, thus assuring that everybody gets health care. So far, so good. This is, in fact, basically how it works today, the difference being that in the Romney model the state's commitment to providing health care for the uninsured is completely open-ended.

Now: the point with the model is not only to assure health care for everyone, but—more importantly—to make sure that everyone has health insurance. So there has to be some kind of stopper in the model in order to prevent people from simply passing up on insurance and then just go get whatever care they need anyway.

To avoid this free-rider problem the Romney model lets the state fine employers if their employees: a) have no health insurance, and b) seek health care without health insurance. But the caveat is that the fine does not kick in from day one—contrary to what one would expect, the state does not send the full bill for an employee's uninsured health care to his employer. Instead, the employee can get free health care on two separate occasions. Upon the third visit to the doctor, the state finally sends a bill to the employer.

And then only if the total sum of free health care that one employer's employees have received, exceeds $50,000.

In other words: a firm with five employees can let its workers go without health insurance, and they can enjoy $10,000 worth of health care each over one year, without any repercussions for the employer.

That is a lot of health care. It is so much, in fact, that the threat of a fine is worth practically nothing.

Consider this. In 2005, the per capita personal health care spending in Massachusetts was $7,200. Some people, obviously, consumed a whole lot more—such as cancer patients, women having difficult births, the severely ill on long term care, etc. But an average healthy person does not consume health care for nearly that amount. Let alone for $50,000.

So that small business owner with five employees is faced with an interesting financial decision. He can buy insurance for his employees at $10,000 each, per year. Or he can let them consume health care for free up to the $50,000 cap and then pay a fine (which will be far less than $50,000 per year).

Will he buy health insurance? *Duh …*

The state is trying to anticipate this free rider problem by adding another regulation. (Isn't it interesting how one government regulation necessitates another regulation….?) If the employees of one employer receive state paid health care more than five times per year, in total, then the state starts sending bills to that employer.

But even that regulation has a caveat (they all do—hence the patchwork of government regulations that we have to put up with!). The state has, as we know, promised to pay health insurance for anyone who cannot afford it. This promise must also extend to employers, right? After all, they are private citizens just like individuals are. Suppose that small business with five employees is working hard to establish itself on a new market. Suppose that it is breaking even without paying the $50,000 in health insurance for its employees. The employees know that the employer is going out of his way to make the business grow, and that they also have to work extra hard to make that happen. They like working for him, there is a strong team spirit at the firm and they know that with a little more success the business will eventually be able to provide them with benefits.

But right now, there just is not enough margin for it.

Here comes the state of Massachusetts. The employer has to buy insurance, or his employees will only have one doctor's visit each per year for free. After that, there will be fines to pay for the state. There might even be other punishments down the road. Will the state ban the business from bidding on state contracts?

What does the business do? Without the Romney model, this small business is free to tell its employees that "we are not offering benefits yet" and it is up to the job seeker to accept or decline the job offer. If benefits is what he is looking for, then he can go get another job with benefits. If not, he'll take the job.

Under the Romney model, the business has no choice. It may have to lay off one of its employees and have the rest work harder without more pay.

Or—the business could claim that it cannot afford to buy insurance and therefore request that the state provides subsidies for its employees' health insurance.

Government subsidies—a cost bomb waiting to go off!

Speaking of state-subsidized health insurance. The Romney model promises low income families a state subsidy toward their health insurance premium. Anyone who makes so little that they are classified as poor will have fully tax-paid insurance (Medicaid). That is no news compared to today. The news is that those who make up to 300 percent of the federal poverty limit will be eligible for subsidized health insurance.

It is easy to see that this may cost taxpayers a whole lot of money. But not one official document provides any credible estimate of how much this subsidy will cost.

Why? Good question! (Is it because lawmakers think that "it's not my money anyway ..."? I would hope not, but it makes you wonder, doesn't it??)

So let us do the job here. We obviously need to find out how many people are actually eligible for the subsidy. We also need to find out how big the subsidy is going to be per eligible person.

The size of the subsidy per individual is quite simple to establish. Since the state "expects" an affordable health insurance to cost $200 per month, we can assume that the state will subsidize the health insurance premium from the first dollar above $200. With an average premium being $833, each eligible family can therefore look forward to a subsidy of $633 per month. Or $7,596 per year.

Now, the question is, how many people will be eligible for that subsidy? Well, first of all, every child in the eligible families will be on Medicaid. That means that their insurance is 100 percent paid for by taxpayers. This cost has been factored in to the (tiny) calculations behind the Massachusetts model.

What they have not calculated with is the amount of people that will be eligible for the $7,596 annual subsidy. And that is too bad, because by rough estimate, some 500,000 Massachusetts families will be eligible for the subsidy.[8] Multiplied by $7,596, this amounts to $3.8 billion per year in tax money.

This cost estimate uses U.S. Census data to proxy family sizes and number of kids per family. It should not be taken as a definitive assessment of the total cost to taxpayers for the subsidy part of the plan. But it shows us that even if this was the only extra cost that the model brought about, the reform would end up costing taxpayers four times more than they have been told.

On top of this, we have all the other cost driving factors: small businesses who know that the fine for not providing insurance is smaller than the cost of the insurance; individuals who make more than 300 percent of FPL but still cannot find an affordable plan …

It is fair to expect that the Massachusetts model will cost taxpayers up to $5 billion, or 500 percent more than official estimates.

This is indeed a problem to the model, and something that a fiscal conservative such as Governor Romney should give serious consideration.

But it should not be taken as a death blow to the model itself. On the contrary, the easiest way for the state to avoid these problems is to: a) remove the state mandates and open their Connector to plans from all across the country, and b) delay the subsidies and the purchase mandate with one year, in order to let the market do its work. If the model works well and the uninsured problem "solves itself" with the help of the market, then the state can simply scrap the rest of the regulations.

Checklist for a national version of the Romney model

To recap, here is a plan for cheaper health insurance without big government:

- Build a national Connector where insurance plans from all states are sold.

- Create a small business pool within the Connector where small businesses get big business leverage. This means better rates and grants them the same rights as big businesses get under their ERISA exemptions.

- Single state registration—so long as a plan has been registered in one state and meets that state's coverage mandates, it can be offered through the national Connector to any resident of the United States

- Delay insurance requirement for individuals—let the free market work for at least three years, and then evaluate if it has done a good job

- <u>Preserve Medicaid for the poor</u> instead of letting it expand into middle class income layers—this way we can actually keep taxes down while letting the free market do its job and keep costs down for all of us

- <u>No price regulations</u>—if the government promotes competition and consumer choice, it will actually do more for health care affordability than artificial price regulations.

With these modifications, the Romney model can in fact become *the health reform of the century*.

BUT ISN'T UNIVERSAL
HEALTH CARE BETTER?

Almost every liberal, and surprisingly many conservatives, would like to see the government run our health care system. Somehow, there is this belief that universal health care is a natural part of a societal evolution. In his 2004 presidential campaign, Senator Kerry hinted that America was backwards compared to other industrialized nations who have universal health care.[9]

Democratic presidential candidates since at least Michael Dukakis have consistently proposed universal health care,[10] and the idea is still very much alive among leading Democrats.[11] A government health monopoly is proposed by 2008 presidential candidate John Edwards[12] as well as by Senator Kerry[13].

But what is it they really want? Beyond the appealing rhetoric about everybody getting all the health care they want—what are the backers of universal health care actually proposing?

It is not entirely easy to answer that question. Most of the pro-government health care suggestions appear to be designed to give the impression of making the candidate look good, more than anything else. There are very few elaborated proposals out there.

The stand-out exception is president Clinton's 1994 plan; the most extensive current proposal for universal health care, presented in California, is a simplified version of the Clinton plan.

President Clinton was candid enough to let the American people know how he was going to finance his proposal. It was good for America that it never became the law of the land, but it was nevertheless a respectable and carefully designed proposal. Today's proponents of universal health should take note. (Of course, an elaborate financing plan would not make their proposals more workable—but it would make them more credible.)

To make matters worse, advocates of socialized health care do not seem to have sorted out the terminology for themselves. We hear about *universal health care, universal health insurance, single payer health insurance, socialized health,* com-

prehensive health coverage ... They all seem to mean the same thing, but at the end of the day they don't.

It is about time that we straighten out the terms and get on top of the debate.

Universal health insurance

The most commonly used word in the government-health debate is **universal**. It is used in **universal health insurance** and means "everyone" as in "everyone has health insurance". The practical meaning is that every legal resident of a state (and illegal, if you are in California) or a country has health insurance.

Let us notice, already here and now, that there are *two important restrictions* on universal health insurance:

- it does *not* guarantee health care to patients without upfront costs, and

- it does *not* provide every conceivable benefit.

In fact, all that universal health insurance means is that every resident *must have* health insurance. Many people who use the term "universal health insurance" mistakenly believe that just because you create universal health insurance, patients pay nothing upfront. But that is not the case. Under universal health insurance there is a law that says that every patient has health insurance—how that health insurance is paid for is another matter. Usually, most of it is paid through taxes, but there are supplemental fees of all kinds that patients themselves must cover in order to get all the health care they need.

The Romney model is, actually, a good example of a universal health insurance system. The key is its individual mandate, which dictates that every resident of Massachusetts must have health insurance.

This all sounds very good, but as we have already seen, requiring individuals to purchase health insurance opens a can of government regulation worms. One regulation leads to a new problem, which is then met with a new regulation ...

As a matter of fact, Massachusetts is a good example of the second restriction on universal health insurance systems that we mentioned above. The second restriction says that universal health systems do not provide all benefits in the world. It is a widespread myth, especially among liberal supporters of universal health insurance, that it is some sort of magic wand that you can swing and all of a sudden everyone gets all the health care they could possibly wish for. This is not true, especially if our definition of "health care" includes such benefits as psychiatrists, psychologists, chiropractors, dentists or opticians. In many countries with universal health insurance people pay dearly for these benefits, on top of what they pay in taxes.[14]

The reason why no universal health insurance system can offer "everything to everyone" is, of course, that no health care is free. For every new benefit that we add to a health plan, more money must be put in to it. That money has to come from somewhere, either our net tax income, or out of our gross income as higher taxes.

For this reason, universal health systems always cap what benefits are mandated. In Massachusetts, the cap consists of the coverage mandates: they dictate the minimum of what a health plan must cover, but thereby they also dictate a *coverage maximum*. No plan has to provide benefits beyond the state's coverage mandates.

This means that if you live in Massachusetts you will have to pay for a long list of health care out of your own pocket—*despite the fact that the Romney model provides universal health insurance*. Here are some examples:

- <u>Autism</u>—if your child is autistic, you will have to pay for therapy and treatment yourself

- <u>Bone mass measurement</u>;

- <u>Chemotherapy</u>—it is not mandatory that health insurance plans in Massachusetts pay for chemotherapy;

- <u>Cleft palate</u>—fixing this can cost a lot of money, and in Massachusetts you will have to pay for it yourself unless you buy an insurance plan that offers extra coverage on top of the state mandates;

- <u>Colorectal cancer screening</u>;

- <u>Dental anesthesia</u>—another costly benefit that is not mandated in Massachusetts;

- <u>Hospice and long term care</u>;

- <u>Pain management specialists</u>;

- <u>Physical therapists</u>.

In defense of the Romney model, we should notice that by not mandating everything, the model leaves it up to consumers to make some health insurance choices. It is also good, as we noticed before, that the model does not introduce a *single payer*. A single payer system is one where all health care is paid for by one single government agency. The Romney model stops short of this—in fact, it is precisely for this reason that it is an interesting alternative to single payer models.

Universal <u>*single payer*</u> *health insurance*

A single payer system is the next step, after universal health insurance. It adds a government agency to the universal coverage, with the sole responsibility of paying for health care. That agency is then the only payer of health care expenses in the state (or the country, if we build a federal system).

The single payer system is the one that most liberals refer to when they talk about universal health insurance. Critics rightfully refer to it as socialized health.

In a single payer system, it is not necessary that health care providers are government employees. In Denmark, e.g., family doctors have their own private practice and get reimbursed from the government health care agency for their patients. However, since the government has a monopoly on paying for insurance, it does not really make a difference whether the doctor is technically self employed or not. So long as his only source of income is what the government provides, he is virtually a government employee anyway. If the government decides to cut reimbursement rates for patients, in order to balance its budget, then the self employed doctor has no choice but to cope with that.

Since the government controls the entire health care budget they can also regulate the number of doctors, specialists, clinics and hospitals in any given area. They can do it indirectly by increasing or decreasing reimbursement rates to health providers—which will make it more or less attractive for, say, an eye doctor to set up a practice in one city as opposed to another. They can also regulate the numbers directly by simply introducing permits for a certain number of specialists and general practitioners.

This type of regulation fills one purpose only, and that is to allow the government to contain health care costs. If the single payer system was put in place to make sure that everyone got the health care they needed, and for no other purpose, then there would be no need to regulate supply of health care.

For the same reason, single payer systems like the Clinton plan and the current California proposal also make it illegal for health care providers to sell their services for private money. If they receive money from the government for the health care that they deliver, they cannot sell care to patients privately on their free time. The idea is to discourage doctors from moonlighting in a private practice, which—the argument goes—would take time and money away from the government's health system.

But what it really means is that the government wants to be able to minimize the number of doctors, to keep costs down, and let the ones they have work extra time instead. Whether or not this is smart on behalf of the government is an open question, to be generous. But this is nevertheless the reason why single payer systems are coupled with a legal ban on private health services (except for the ones that the government does not pay for).

This leads to supply rationing—also known as waiting lists—in virtually every part of the health care system. In every country with a single payer system, the government's efforts to keep costs down take charge over the same government's promise to provide good, timely health care to its people. Patients in Canada, Britain and Sweden, to mention only a few, can bear witness of this, and how they have no choice but to cope with the situation as best they can.

Are these excessive regulations a price worth paying? Should we put up with the waiting lists, because the moral goal with universal access to health care is higher?

Superficially, yes. Nothing could be more compassionate than having taxpayers share the bill for all our health care. That way, nobody is allegedly left without health care because they cannot afford it.

But single payer systems always cost more and give less than private insurance. This arises from the inevitable inefficiency in all government operations.

Another, often forgotten, dimension of the single payer system is that its cost containment efforts make it unprofitable to develop new, expensive medical technology. Other technologies and treatment methods that are not quite familiar to our medical profession may never get a chance to prove themselves.

Acupuncture is a good example. In California's single payer bill introduced last year, called SB-840, it says explicitly that the state will only pay for medical treatment that is determined to have "medical indication" by the state's chief medical officer. If acupuncture would be introduced under such a system, the state would not pay for acupuncture treatment. At the time when it was first brought to Western societies, it was frowned upon by the medical establishment. In countries with single payer health insurance the governments relied on their "chief medical officers" and decided that acupuncture had no medical value and should therefore not be paid for by taxpayers.

Today acupuncture is widely accepted. California is one of eleven states with a coverage mandate for acupuncturists. But the only reason why acupuncture is an established method in our health care system is because medical professionals introduced it into a free market system where people had a chance to choose for themselves what treatment methods they want, and what they do not want.

Entrepreneurs take chances, hoping to create a niche where they can make good money and be successful. Some fail, others succeed. Doctors can learn and practice new treatment methods that may not be entirely accepted by the majority of their colleagues. They can then prove that those methods work, and thereby bring an entire field in health care forward.

That is how we are introduced to new ideas. Thanks to a free market, new ideas in medicine are brought to patients faster than under a government monopoly. A free health insurance market allows consumers to choose what health benefits they want covered. Insurance providers compete with different benefits packages. If a lot of us want acupuncture covered, then it will be covered by a lot of insurance plans.

A chief medical officer in a single payer system can very well be encouraged not to accept new medical procedures not because they have no "medical indication", but because they cost too much.

In fact, California's SB-840 bill explicitly says that health care expenditures must not grow faster than the sum of state GDP growth and population growth. Anything that will drive costs higher will be left unpaid for by the system. It really does not matter how good and revolutionary the new medical procedure is. According to SB-840 there are no exceptions to the budget cap.

Sounds cynical? Indeed it does. But the fact of the matter is that this is what the California bill suggests. Centralized, bureaucratic control has these consequences.

But the problem gets worse. In a free market system new, expensive technologies and methods are first applied in the high end of the market. Over time the costs fall and the new med-tech and treatment methods trickle down to become part of everyday health care.

There is nothing strange with this—it works the same way in all markets. Safety systems in cars were first introduced as high cost options on luxury cars. Today, even compact cars with modest price stickers come equipped with valuable techniques like electronic stability systems and anti-lock brakes.

This is how our lives get better. Those who invent new technologies earn their first profits by selling it at high price, to pay off the expensive development costs. Over time we all benefit.

Under a government health monopoly, things are different. There is no high end market for expensive, new treatment methods or cutting edge medical technology. Decisions on what med-tech hospitals and clinics should use are exclusively in the hands of a few government bureaucrats. If under a single payer system a private hospital (that gets all its money from the state) buys expensive new technology without approval from the state's chief medical officer, then it is not going to get reimbursed.

Obviously, knowing this the hospital will not acquire the new technology in the first place.

The single payer system discourages innovation and encourages status quo.

And it does not stop at excluding new medical procedures or new technology. The government can even choose to deny mortally ill patients existing treatment because it would cost too much to treat them.

Consider the case of Mr. Lesley Burke, a British man with a terrible disease. He felt it necessary to take the National Health Service, NHS, to court to assure that he would receive certain treatments in the final days of his life.[15] Mr. Burke …

> … has a progressive neurological disease that may one day deprive him of the ability to swallow. If that happens, Burke wants to receive food and water through a tube. Knowing that Britain's National Health Service (NHS) rations care, Burke sued to ensure that he will not be forced to endure death by dehydration against his wishes.

He had good reasons to do so:

> According to National Health Service treatment guidelines, doctors, rather than patients or their families, have the final say about providing or withholding care.

The reason for this is, of course, that Britain's tax paid health care system has to comply with a painfully tight budget cap. When patients demand more health care than the government has budgeted for, doctors and budget administrators let budget considerations override medical decisions.

All in the name of cost containment.

Nonsense? Unfortunately not. This is a harsh reality in single payer systems. Mr. Burke is not a fictional character. He is a living, breathing man, and he lost his lawsuit. The NHS successfully made the case that the pain that he would suffer toward the end of his life would not be severe enough to motivate spending money on him.

With the firm, tight budget cap in California's SB-840, Californians can look forward to similar experiences unless Governor Schwarzenegger can prevail in his opposition to the bill.

Comprehensive Health Insurance

Another term that is being thrown around by those who want more government in health care is **comprehensive health insurance**. Theoretically, this would mean something less ambitious than *universal* health insurance: either most people have "universal" insurance, or all people have limited but legally guaranteed insurance.

In practice, though, comprehensive health insurance is just a smoke screen for universal health insurance. A lot of times when politicians talk about "comprehensive" insurance, they are doing so deliberately because they know that "universal" health insurance is unpopular.

A good example is Verla Insko, state legislator from Orange County in North Carolina. In April 2006 she told a state legislative committee on health care that the committee ought to recommend *comprehensive* health coverage precisely because, she said, people will respond negatively to the term "universal".[16]

So in order to deceive voters and get what she wants, Ms. Insko tricks them into believing that she really wants something else. As harsh as it sounds, the only way to characterize Ms. Insko is that she is disingenuous and deceitful. She is purposely undermining people's faith in their elected officials and has no respect for the will of the people. It is, of course, ultimately up to the voters of Orange County, North Carolina to decide how far they want to be deceived, but since Ms. Insko is deliberately blowing smoke screens, they will first have to acknowledge her deception.

That is a big step for all of us, and it does not exactly increase our respect for politicians.

Overall, of course, the term "comprehensive" is used honestly and with the best of intentions. So long as we can cut through the smoke screens and tell genuine arguments from the deceptive ones, we can stay make those good intentions deliver.

Next, let us take a look at the morale behind universal, single payer health care. Many people believe that it is so ethically right that we should be able to put up with even significant shortcomings in the system.

Should we?

BUT HOW CAN YOU DENY ANYBODY HEALTH CARE??

A lot of people support universal, single payer health insurance because they genuinely believe that it will give all of us better health care. That is a false belief, of course, but it is nevertheless a respectable position that deserves recognition and a good answer.

But there is also a strong moral dimension in the argument for a single payer system. It is undoubtedly an appealing idea that everyone should have all the health care they could ever need.

Who can disagree with *that*?

Well, the fact of the matter is that nobody disagrees with that view. With the exception of complete wing nuts, we all want the best for all our fellow humans.

We are Americans. It is in our blood stream to be generous and caring, and we *are* generous and caring. We are the most compassionate people on Earth—no matter what your college professors told you …! ;=)

So the issue here is not who is the most compassionate and caring among us. The issue is instead how we best transform that compassion and care into real life, actionable policy.

The only way to really evaluate the moral argument for single payer health insurance is to see if it can actually deliver the compassion and care that it claims it can. That is almost a no-brainer, but as we will see later, a lot of the plans for universal, single payer health insurance lack the substance to deliver better health care. They talk the talk but don't walk the walk.

When people make the case for universal health care without being able to back it up with real, actionable policy—including numbers that makes it a credible proposal—then their moral arguments are little more than verbal vanity.

If a proposal for single payer health insurance—such as SB-840 in California—can credibly argue that it will indeed deliver on its moral pledge, then it has passed the verbal vanity test. If not, we better ask the politicians behind the proposal some really hard questions.

The first and foremost reason why most arguments for single payer systems do not pass the verbal vanity test is that they fail to realize that most existing single payer systems *deny people health care*. It makes me uneasy to see how this simple fact is ignored over and over again by lawmakers and other influential people who propose single payer systems. Our next chapter will present evidence of this denial of care, evidence that anyone who wants single payer health insurance must address.

To pass the verbal vanity test, they must explain what they intend to do differently than the systems that they so often refer to as their role models. They must explain how they can look at Canada without seeing the waiting lists; they must explain how they can look at Britain without seeing cases like Mr. Burke's; they must explain how Sweden can be held in such high esteem when in reality they ration health care far beyond human dignity.

They have to explain all this—or their proposals will be nothing more than verbal vanity.

Single payer systems face steep moral challenges

Health care rationing is the biggest moral challenge to backers of single payer systems. Their model is destined to fare worse then a free market system. In a very tangible way, this means less care, worse care and in many cases no care at all—and for whatever health care that we would get, we would pay more than we do today.

Despite all this, many of us are willing to accept the shortcomings of the single payer model, simply because its superficial moral appeal is so strong. The natural question to ask is, of course, whether a free market based health care system is at all better. Does it not leave people behind? If someone simply cannot afford health insurance, does the free market system even care?

Of course it does. Or, more correctly, *we* care. First of all, we already have Medicaid, which was created to provide health insurance for the poor. Medicaid has expanded a bit too far in most states, and made private insurance more expensive (yes, it's true!) but there is nothing wrong with the basic idea. If we take care of Medicaid and make sure that it is focused on the poor, then we have a good safety net for the really needy. Then we can concentrate our efforts on making the free market work well.

One of the most widespread myths of today is that a free health insurance market will only benefit the rich. But that is not true. The people who would really be in trouble in a single payer system in America are families with low and moderate income. They will be trapped in a system that gives worse health care than they get today.

The rich, on the other hand, will escape the waiting lists, and denials of care, and fly somewhere where there are private clinics. That is exactly what is going on in Canada. Rich Canadians fly south to American hospitals when their single payer system lets them down. Regular families are cannot afford to do that. They are stuck with whatever health care the government provides—or fails to provide.

A moral counter-argument to this point would be: "But let's tax the rich more, so we can get more resources to put in to our single payer system. That way the regular families will benefit and the rich might even have to stay at home and share in the experience."

But is there really enough rich people to tax for that purpose? No, there isn't. And herein lies the second moral challenge to the single payer system. While it claims to benefit low income families, it will inevitably come to tax them a whole lot more than the rich.

Yes.

Virtually every country with a single payer health insurance system has maxed out its taxation of the rich and has had to start raising taxes on low income families. This is the only way that they can get enough funds for their health care system. America still makes the rich pay most of the taxes—we still have a progressive tax system—while countries like Netherlands, Denmark, Sweden and Finland have regressive tax systems. In other words: tax systems that make low income families pay a disproportionately high share of the taxes.[17]

It is particularly interesting to see that Sweden has a regressive tax system. The country has been held in high esteem by liberals for decades as a role model to America. But I seriously doubt that they would like to import the Swedish tax system to pay for all the entitlement programs that liberals want—such as a single payer health insurance system.

The lowest paid 30 percent of Sweden's families earn 10.9 percent of all income, but they pay 12 percent of all taxes.

By contrast, the highest paid 30 percent make 53 percent of the income and pay almost exactly the same share of taxes.

This is important. It shows what happens to an economy when we start relying on the government for everything and anything—especially health care.

Let us compare Sweden to U.S. data. America's lowest paid three deciles earn 9.5 percent of all income, but they only pay 6.8 percent of the taxes. The highest paid three deciles, on the other hand, make 56 percent of all income but pay 64 percent of all taxes.

The Canadian numbers are not as bad as the Swedish ones, mostly because Canada has not gone to such extremes as Sweden has in terms of building a full-fledged welfare state. But low income families in Canada are still burdened with higher taxes than they would be in America.

If a U.S. state like California actually creates a full scale single payer system, it will by necessity have to imitate many parts of the Canadian—or even Swedish—tax system. Otherwise, they won't be able to pay for all that health care through taxes. They also have the problem that if they raise taxes on the rich and wealthy far above other states, they will see an unprecedented flight of people and money out of the state.

Bottom line: the single payer system looks good on paper, but cannot deliver on its moral promises. It gives less care to the middle class, and low income families, while asking them all to pay more for that same rationed care.

No matter how hard we try, a single payer system does not stand up to moral scrutiny. It cannot deliver on its promise of "free" gold plated health care for everyone.

Perhaps we will get there some time in the future, when we are no longer bound by our society's scarcity of resources. Maybe some day we will have Star Trek-style "replicators" that can create just about anything, even surgeon robots ...

But right here, right now, the facts of reality are that we have to opt for the health care system that *actually* delivers as much as possible to all of us. The only system capable of doing that is one that is based on free markets. We can never create a perfect health care system, but we can get as close to perfection as possible. And the real indicator of how close we are to perfection is how good health care the poor and the middle class can get.

Today, in America, the single payer system cannot pass the verbal vanity test. Our current system is far from perfect, but it is a much better foundation for improvement than any single payer system would ever be.

Free markets and generosity

Contrary to the stereotypical image of a Capitalist society that is often promoted on our college campuses, Capitalism actually promotes compassion, generosity and care for those in need. Charitable giving is one of the most admirable institutions in America. It is a core feature of our society and supports institutions that help the poor and needy. It keeps the government from putting bureaucrats in charge of welfare programs.

Charitable giving and direct involvement in social issues build strong, lasting institutions with personal responsibility on both sides. A free market economy with low taxes and limited government promotes more of this. The Charities Aid Foundation in Britain has shown that people in countries with low taxes and limited government are more generous and give more to charity than people in high tax countries with big welfare states.

Together, Medicaid and charitable giving create a good safety net for the neediest among us. With a well working free market system we can assure that only an absolute minimum of our fellow citizens will ever need Medicaid or the help of charitable institutions. We do not have a well working free market in health care today, but we have a good foundation to build on. I am convinced that the combination of a better free market system, a limited and focused Medicaid and a strong voluntary sector is all we need.

Bottom line: more economic and individual freedom is a better way to good health care for everybody, than more government. It means that we have to accept inequalities—differences is a better term—but if we can get past that and see what the free market can do for us, then we will actually be able to make some real improvements to our health care system.

WE'RE SORRY, ALL DOCTORS ARE BUSY TREATING OTHER PATIENTS ...

Time now for the biggest challenge to the friends of single payer systems: waiting lists.

Of all the universal, single payer health insurance bills that I discuss in this book, not one—not a single one—discusses the waiting list problem. There are few things that can make a politician look dishonest, but this is one of them.

What makes the waiting list problem so dangerous is that it appears to be deceptively small. Hey, all it means is that you have to wait a little longer to see the doctor, right?

Well, it's a whole lot more than that. Any single payer proponent who dismisses the waiting list problem as a minor issue—or refuses to discuss it at all—is arrogantly ignorant about the true nature of single payer health care.

Waiting lists are not just numbers on a piece of paper. They are very real, so real, in fact that they can literally be lethal.

Yes, waiting lists kill people.

Fortunately, the death toll in most countries with single payer health care is so small that it does not affect longevity or other aggregated health data. But that does not help those who die from curable cancer diseases because they are not allowed to see a doctor in time. (Besides, we should not have to wait until people start dying in large numbers in countries with single payer systems, before America's single payer advocates start paying attention to the waiting list problem.)

For a long time, I have believed that single payer advocates do not talk about the waiting list problem simply because they do not have time to sit down and analyze the problem. I imagined that if only they had the chance to study the issue a little bit more, they would eventually come up with a decent idea on how to avoid importing that problem when they import the single payer model itself.

Well, they have had enough time, have they not? They have had so many presidential candidates—from Dukakis to Kerry—who have been promoting single payer health insurance, that it is about time for them to address the waiting list problem.

But they still do not care about it. It is frightening, quite frankly, for someone like me who has seen the waiting list problem from the inside, to watch the aggressive Democratic push for a single payer system. I realize that they simply do not care about the waiting list problem.

They pretend that it does not exist.

Verbal vanity again.

Therefore, since they do not want to discuss the problem, we will do it here instead. And the best place to start is Canada. They are fighting a constant, uphill battle against health care rationing, a battle that they have, of course, brought upon themselves.

In 2005 that battle was taken all the way up to the Canadian Supreme Court. In June that year, the Court ruled that Canada's universal health insurance system violated each Canadian's right to "life and personal security, inviolability and freedom".[18] The reason was very simple: regular Canadians had to wait to see a doctor for so long that their health and even lives were in jeopardy.

In other words: waiting lists kill people.

No American would accept the waits that the Canadians have to put up with. For a simple MRI you have to wait almost 18 weeks.[19] If you need to see a medical specialist, you have to wait for an average of eight weeks and five days. Some specialists have much longer waiting lists.

But then, of course, you have to wait to see your general practitioner first. The Canadian system does not allow patients to see a specialist without a referral.[20]

Some waits are just agonizing. Canadians who have been diagnosed with cancer have to wait for three weeks to see an oncologist, and then another three weeks for treatment.[21] For all of us who have experienced deadly cancer in our families, that is long enough.

Cynically speaking (and I really don't want to be cynical about this, but sometimes it is inevitable) a Canadian cancer patient is among the "luckier" ones in Canada. He will certainly not feel better knowing that others have to wait a whole lot longer, but the truth is that those six weeks are short by comparison:

Total wait to see a specialist and receive treatment

	Referral	See specialist	Treatment	Total days
Cancer patient	Sept 1	Sept 22	Oct 14	42
Eye doctor	Sept 1	Dec 17	March 2	183
Orthopedist	Sept 1	Dec 22	June 8	286

Of course, these waiting times are psychologically stressful and means serious financial trouble to many people. Many of them cannot work or have to limit their work days to part time. For elderly people who are retired and in bigger need to be mobile, an untreated medical condition can be a life changing experience to the worse, with social isolation and poorer general health as a result.

As we have already noted, Canadians with money simply escape these waiting lists and fly south to American hospitals. It was with this reality in mind that the Canadian Supreme Court ruled against the single payer system. Government run health care was putting people's lives and freedom in jeopardy, and that had to stop.

Now American liberals want the same system here, and if they cannot get it nationally, they will push for it in California, Connecticut, Hawaii, Kansas, Maine, Maryland, Missouri, New Hampshire, New York, North Carolina, Vermont, Wisconsin ...

Another thing that is frightening about this waiting list problem is that once we have it, it is almost impossible to get rid of it. There are a number of reasons for this, but one is in the nature of the single payer system itself. The route to universal health care is a one way street. Canada is once again a case in point: despite the 2005 Supreme Court ruling, the situation is still virtually unchanged, with the same long waiting lists and wealthy patients flying south to get away from it.

There is a simple reason for this. Once we have eradicated the free health insurance market, we will be paying such high taxes that we will be unable to afford private health insurance. In other words: if we try to re-introduce a private health insurance market, very few people will have any margins left to purchase those plans. Since very few people can buy private insurance while still paying huge taxes for a dysfunctional government run health system, insurance providers will be hard pressed to offer low cost plans. The risk is simply too high.

In short: once we have universal, single payer health insurance, we are stuck with it.

Canadian politicians have apparently realized this. Despite their Supreme Court's ruling they are not exactly leaping to change their poorly working, expensive system. At best, they float proposals to cap waiting times. But as this story in the *Toronto Star* shows,[22] such caps are nothing more than promises:

> Federal Health Minister Tony Clement says he doesn't know when patients will see promised guarantees on medical wait times, but his Ontario counterpart bets it'll be a while. "A time frame of a few years would be more appropriate," George Smitherman told reporters yesterday at a conference on the future of medicare.... "I don't have an exact date," said Clement, whose government made the guarantees one of its five key promises in the last election because of concerns Canadians are waiting too long for treatment.... Under the guarantee, patients would get treatment close to home within what medical experts deem to be a reasonable period of time or be sent elsewhere at government expense.

The situation is hardly better in other countries with single payer systems. In 2001, 38 percent of British patients in need of any type of elective surgery had to wait, on average, more than four months before they could be treated.[23] How much more than four months is not reported.

It was 23 percent in Australia.

It gets worse when we look at specific types of surgery. Spanish patients in need of orthopedic surgery had to wait more than a year. The same applied to Spanish women waiting for hysterectomy, which is a serious procedure used to cure very painful or dangerous medical conditions.

Needless to say, a one year wait for something of that magnitude is a very stressful and agonizing experience.

What few people seem to know is that the United States is recognized internationally as *having no waiting list problem*.[24] A telling example: patients in need of hip replacement. According to the Paris-based OECD, a big international economic research institution, American hip replacement patients do not have to wait longer than medically reasonable. By contrast, in Australia, Denmark, England, Finland, Netherlands, Norway and Spain waiting times are excessive, ranging anywhere from 100 to 250 days. For a September 1 referral, a 250 day wait means surgery on May 8 the following year.

Hip replacement patients are often elderly who become immobile with a bad hip. Therefore, excessive waiting periods causes social isolation as well as serious health problems and may even lead to pre-mature death.

A Swedish daily, *Sundsvalls Tidning*, recently published a story that illustrates the agony that rationed health care can cause, precisely with reference to elderly with hip problems. It is about an 82-year-old man and his battle with a government health monopoly that creates waiting lists in order to keep health care costs down:[25]

> The hip got dislodged over and over again, he went in and out the hospital, had to wait ten months for a new surgery contracted [a serious bacterial infection while at the hospital]./.../82-year-old Eric Lindahl himself thinks that incompetence explains his situation. He also thinks that he has been met with indifference by doctors./.../Already before the replacement of his right-side prosthetic hip joint in January last year, Mr. Lindahl became aware that the procedure could become complicated. The prosthetic hip joint had been replaced several times before and during the past six months his problems [with the hip joint] had accelerated. Soon after the replacement surgery he started having severe pains, which turned out to be caused by the fact that the femur had been cracked [sic!] during the procedure./.../But the real problems started when Mr. Lindahl's hip joint got dislodged. It happened time and time again during the spring and summer [of 2006]. Mr. Lindahl went to the hospital several times, med a number of different doctors and claims that he unsuccessfully tried to reach his surgeon, Dr. Lennart Bengtson, head of the orthopedic clinic. He was promised a new surgery on the hip/.../. During the fall he called [the orthopedic clinic] numerous times to get an appointment for the new surgery. A new doctor was assigned [by the hospital bureaucracy] and he concluded that the prosthetic hip joint was too short. Surgery was done in December. Mr. Lindahl was discharged from the hospital but the wound after the surgery did not heal. Toward the end of December he was taken in to the hospital again./.../Mr. Lindahl had contracted an infection with multi-resistant bacteria. He was originally scheduled for treatment at the clinic for infectuous diseases but that clinic was closed due to [stomach flu]./ .../'I want the people in charge to know that we do not have health care worth mentioning in cases like this' Mr. Lindahl says.

There are countless experiences like this from single payer systems, and the waiting list problem stretches across the entire spectrum of medical specialties. In all these instances the American system outperforms single payer systems. American men who need prostate surgery can be lucky that they do not live in Australia, Finland, Netherlands or Norway. While American prostate patients get surgery in time that is medically acceptable, their peers in these other countries have to wait up to three months—a very long time in this context.

Patients in need cataract surgery in America have no waiting list problem, but in Australia, England, Finland and Sweden they have to wait 200 days on average. That is March 19, with a September 1 referral. If you are referred for general eye surgery on September 1, your operation may be as far away as April 14 the next spring.

These examples should be bad enough to make us think twice before we promote a single payer system in America—or in any one state.

But it does not stop here. Some European countries make the Canadian waiting lists look humane. Once again: this happens because once the health system goes bad, there is no stopping it from going catastrophic. Once the health care socialists have it their way in America, we will end up like Canada, at the very least. But we could just as well plunge to the levels of England. Not to mention Sweden, where cancer patients are dying of curable diseases and hospitals in the nation's capital have to send complicated births abroad, all because of an inefficient government monopoly that operates under a severe cost containment regime.

The human suffering among people who are forced to wait for months—sometimes more than a year—is horrific. But the health horrors from single payer systems do not stop at elective surgery and non-emergency care. They even extend into the ER.

On December 3, 2006, the Swedish daily *Aftonbladet* published a story about a three-year-old boy who got sick from a regular stomach condition.[26] His parents grew concerned and sought help at the local ER. It deserves to be noted that this ER was not at some rural hospital with limited resources. It was at one of Sweden's top university hospitals, supposedly well equipped and staffed with enough skilled medical professionals to provide safe, reliable health care.

Because he had lost a lot of body fluids—which you do with a stomach condition—the little boy needed intra-venal liquid supply. His parents came to the ER so that he could get that, be stabilized and get well enough to go home again.

The problem was, nobody at the ER had time to attend to him. Over and over again his parents tried to get the attention of the ER staff, but the hours went by and nothing happened. With an intra-venal supply of fluids he would have been fine, but since he did not get the little help he needed, his body could not fight the stomach infection.

Gradually, he succumbed to the infection. After three hours his pulse dropped dramatically. The initially harmless infection had reached his heart. The ER staff eventually responded, but it was too late.

Two hours later—after a total of five hours in the ER—he was pronounced dead.

Another news story from the same newspaper tells of a man who came to see the local doctor because he felt unusually tired.[27] The doctor told him to go home and quit smoking. This did not help. The man still felt unusually tired and came back to the doctor. He was dismissed as imagining things.

Over the next year the man came back a total of 14 times, feeling worse every time. Each time the doctor told him he was imagining and denied him even a simple blood test. Even when he had blood in his urine, the doctor refused him a thorough examination.

The doctor's motivation—and this is an actual quote from the newspaper article—was that the government-run, tax-funded health care system needed to contain its costs.

The man's son eventually took him to a hospital in a bigger town, three hours away, where he was finally tested the way he should have been tested from the start. It turned out the man had cancer. But not only that: over the course of the year when the cost containing doctor denied him care, the cancer had grown so bad that there was nothing left to do.

It would be wrong to cast all the blame for this on the doctor who refused him care. First of all, since the Swedish health care system is run by the government, a patient—or his family—cannot sue the system for malpractice. (The Clinton plan intended to practically eliminate malpractice lawsuits.) Therefore, there is, technically, no legal way to make the doctor pay for refusing to treat him.

But more importantly, the doctor himself is a government employee. As such, his loyalty lies with his employer, not with his patients. A doctor that has his own clinic and is reimbursed by private insurance companies on behalf of his patients has an entirely different responsibility. He answers to his patients—if they do not like what he does, he goes out of business.

The government, especially in this Swedish case, would not find that the doctor has done anything wrong. Why? Because he has met their obligations to contain the cost of health care at his government-run clinic.

It is the same with waiting lists. Quite frankly, governments do not care about waiting lists if at the same time their single payer systems contain costs and balance their budgets. The Canadian Supreme Court's ruling is exceptional in this context. As we have seen, it is also *by no means* a guarantee that litigation can in fact improve a single payer system.

Rationed health care vs. the uninsured?

It matters to tell these horror stories, because they put flesh and blood on the price that we all will have to pay for a single payer system. But some would rightfully object that while these stories are frightening, and the suffering is simply inhumane, there are tens of millions of Americans who suffer today because they have no insurance at all.

That is a very important objection. But first of all, I am not telling these stories to try to play one-up-man-ship with advocates of universal health care. I am not trying to say that the suffering of millions of people on waiting lists in single payer system countries are worse than the suffering of millions of Americans without health insurance.

My point is, instead, that we should not cause one problem while trying to fix another. The suffering of someone on a waiting list is bad as it is. The testimonies from single payer systems are bad in themselves. We do not need to compare the suffering of people who have insurance but cannot get health care (single payer) to the suffering of people who do not have insurance at all (our imperfect system).

People who are or have been without health insurance know the stress that this causes. In a similar way, people who have been denied health care under a single payer system because the government monopoly cannot afford to provide it are subject to tremendous stress. I have experienced both. I would not want to compare them in any other way than that they both cause tremendous stress, emotionally as well as financially.

The questions we ask ourselves are often similar: Will my condition get worse because I cannot get treatment now? If I am so sick that I cannot work, and I have to wait for months for treatment, how will I pay my bills? How can I get around and see friends and family with this medical condition untreated?

Another side to the single payer system is that while it helps the uninsured to some health care, it brings rationing and denials of care to everyone else. It would be a bad mistake to create a single payer system to help the uninsured and see the deterioration of health care for the rest of the population as a price worth paying. That is just as wrong as trying to determine whether a person on a nine-month long waiting list for orthopedic surgery is suffering more, or less, than a person who cannot get surgery now because he has no health insurance.

Any health care reform that leaves some people worse off, in order to improve health care for others, is a bad reform.

The best way to avoid this is to improve the free market system. Please see the Way Forward chapter at the end of this book for a more elaborate discussion on how to do that. Before we get there, though, we need to talk a little bit more about a third drawback of the single payer system.

We know that it means higher taxes. We also known that it means health care rationing and agonizing waiting lists.

What is little known is that single payer health care is also inefficient.

"SINGLE PAYER SYSTEMS ARE MORE COST EFFICIENT ..."

... or so they say. Many advocates of universal health care refer to studies that show that a government monopoly spends less on administration than a private system. Their argument is usually based on some common sense idea that it is better to have one bureaucracy for making decisions, processing insurance claims and ordering medicine, than to have many different ones.

There is some evidence to back up this claim. The advocacy group Physicians for a National Health Plan[28] refers to several studies according to which a socialized system would make health care administration cheaper. The typical savings are around 3–5 percent of total health spending.

Assuming four percent on average, this means that a national single payer system would save $80 billion per year. In California it would amount to $5 billion, or $224 per working age Californian.

Such savings are certainly desirable. In fact, a superficial look at a socialized health system certainly gives the impression of efficiency and streamlined administration. It seems like they have done a great job at slimming down waste and focused resources on treating patients.

The problem is that you can only save so much on administration. The health care organization still has to make a lot of decisions—administrative decisions. At every hospital, somebody has to keep track of medical records, order supplies, write schedules for the staff, write checks, send bills, keep track of how laws and regulations are adhered to. Someone has to order food, make a budget, assess the quality of everything from bathroom cleaning to the care that nurses and physicians provide ...

No organization can be slimmed to such a degree that these decisions are not made. Nor can you put just anyone at a desk and expect them to be good administrators. The best people to make most of administrative decisions are—professional administrators. And you have to compensate them accordingly.

This is where I begin to question the credibility of those who say that we will save big time on administration in a single payer system. Most of those sweeping cost cut promises come across as little more than political hype.

Many of these studies look at how big the administration staff is in health care, compared to the number of medical professionals. They also look at how much of a budget is itemized as administration, vs. health care itself. These methods make a health care system like the Swedish one look incredibly efficient, and the reason is—simply—that the government has fired a lot of administrators in their relentless attempts to contain health care costs.

But they have not removed the need to make decisions. So someone else has to make them. That someone else is a medical professional. A nurse or a doctor.

A case in point is the Swedish county of Gavleborg. (Since Physicians for a National Health Plan refer to Sweden as having a good single payer system, it is only fair that we go there and have a look.) In Sweden, the health care system is administered by the counties: they own the hospitals, hire the staff and pay all expenses with taxes that they collect from county residents.

So also in Gavleborg.

Of course, the Swedish counties also engage in cost containment. For a long time now they have gone out of their way, every year, to keep health care costs down. One method that is widely practiced is to reduce the administrative staff to an absolute minimum (and the some). In Gavleborg, e.g, the result has been that medical professionals—nursing assistants, nurses, physicians—have to fill in where the administrators left off as they were fired.

So the medical professionals are now spending up to 70 percent of their work time on administration, away from patients.[29]

Yes, up to *70 percent*. Of an eight our shift, they spend five hours and 36 minutes on administration. *Away from patients.*

But how can this look like efficient, streamlined administration??

The answer is simple: a nurse is, by definition, a medical professional. It is assumed that everything she does is caring for and treating patients. Studies of administration costs typically make the unsubstantiated assumption that a nurse does what a nurse is trained to do. So when a nurse does administrative work, the studies report her as actually caring for patients.

It is a no-brainer that patients suffer when medical professionals are assigned to desk jobs. What looks like a nice efficiency gain on the input side (more nurses and doctors per 100 employees at every hospital) ends up as an efficiency loss on the output side (less time for patients per 100 nurses and doctors).

This is not just a theory. It is harsh reality. The drop in output efficiency is well documented. Three researchers at the European Central Bank showed this in a study in 2003.[30] A typical socialized health system delivers less health care per dollar put in to it, than the American health system.

In cold, hard cash: for the health care that costs us $100, many Europeans have to pay $112.

Contrary to what many proponents of universal health care say, their model is *less* efficient.

Let us now recall what Physicians for a National Health Plan said: single payer systems save 3–5 percent on administration. OK? That means some $4 per $100 spent on health care.

We know by now how we achieve that efficiency gain: we lay off administrators and assume that medical professionals only do medically professional work. We save $4 per $100 spent.

Since the administrative work per se has not shrunk, there will be a cost in the other end in the form of a drainage of the work hours of medical professionals. So very same cuts in administration shows up in the other end as a loss in output. That loss, $12 per $100 spent, is a little bit bigger than the initial efficiency gain. Three times bigger, to be exact.

So—*for every dollar that the single payer system saves on more efficient administration, it loses four dollars in lost health care output.*

I know that this goes squarely against what we are commonly being told. We hear over and over again that our American health system is so wasteful and inefficient. But facts are facts, and supporters of universal health care rarely check theirs. It is almost as though they assume that their position is so much more ethical that it does not need more fact-checking.

Again—their arguments do not pass the verbal vanity test.

Let me once again point out that I do not believe that our health system is perfect. Far from it. Low income families who make too much for Medicaid and too little to buy their own insurance, go uninsured. That alone is a clear signal that we have a great deal of work left to do. While only about 15 million of the 45 million uninsured Americans belong to this group, they are still 15 million too many. (The rest are either eligible for Medicaid but have not enrolled, or make enough money to buy insurance themselves, but choose not to.)[31]

But wasting money on a government health monopoly to help this group is like crossing the river to find water. We can achieve a whole lot more in terms of good health care for all, by strengthening the free market. It takes *a lot of hard work*—by legislators, by our governors, our president, but also by us as consumers, voters, patients and taxpayers. We have to educate ourselves, learn to separate good ideas from bad and vote with that in mind.

What matters is that we all understand that there is no better way, and there is no magic wand that we can swing and—*voila!*—the problem is gone. Many of those who want single payer health care seem to believe that a government monopoly is that magic wand.

It is not.

But wait—speaking of efficiency: is it not true that we Americans are paying a lot more for the same health outcomes as others? What about all these people who say that they live at least as long in Europe as we do here in America, and that they pay less than we do, per capita, for health care?

It is tempting to accept this seductive argument without hesitation. After all, who can argue with facts like life expectancy?

This argument is misguided at best, disingenuous at worst. The fact is correct—some countries with socialized health care have longer life expectancy than America—but that does not in any way imply that a single payer system is better than our system.

There is a well concealed false premise behind this argument. Anyone who claims that, e.g., Sweden's higher longevity shows that a single payer system is better, is in fact assuming that most of the health care we consume has to do with life and death.

It is as though almost every decision a medical professional makes will determine whether or not a patient lives to see the next day.

That is of course not true, not for a second. Most health care has to do with treating infections, prescribing drugs, fixing twisted ankles, removing molds ... Other treatments are more complicated, such as hip joint replacement or ear bone implants—complicated surgical jobs but rarely if ever something that will make a difference of life and death to the patient.

If anything, the life-and-death difference between the current American system and a single payer system would tip the other way. It does not, but we also know that socialized health systems make patients wait unacceptably long for treatment. There are rare cases where people actually die from having to wait too long for treatment. Those are so few that they do not change the longevity statistics—something we should be very grateful for, of course.

In any case, the differences in longevity between the United States and some countries with single payer health insurance do not depend on what health system we have. They have to do much more with lifestyle choices than anything else. For one, Danes—who like tobacco, alcohol and fat food—live noticeably shorter than Norwegians, and the countries have almost identical health systems.

The utilitarian dictator—enforcing efficiency in socialized health care

We have already seen that single payer systems fail to deliver on their high pitch morale. But there is a deeper moral problem in those systems, a problem that is perhaps even more serious than the health rationing problem. And this one, single payer advocates strenuously avoid talking about.

It is the utilitarian dictator.

Here is how it works. In order to keep costs down, health politicians and bureaucrats choose not to treat many medical conditions at all. Instead, they concentrate on those where there is the biggest gain from treatment. The gain is defined in terms of utility. The question that guides their choices is: how many QALYs, quality adjusted life years, will I produce if I treat Jack vs. if I treat Jill? The answer determines whether the tax funded, single payer system will treat a patient, or not.

Please note that Jack and Jill have no say in this. They both want treatment, and they both say—rightly so—that they will be infinitely happier once their condition has been treated. But that is not relevant. Instead, the government takes over and determines who—Jack or Jill—will experience the most utility from being treated.

The utilitarian dictator has gone to work. Or, to quote Jane M Orient, writing for *The Freeman* in December 2006: "at some point on the QALY scale, visible to experts, the value of a life becomes negative".

Remember Mr. Burke, the English patient we talked about earlier? This is how he lost his court case. The government's utilitarian dictator—in reality some tax paid bureaucrat—made the case that Mr. Burke would not experience enough QALYs from the treatment he wanted. Instead, the money should be spent on someone else who would experience a lot more QALYs for the same amount.

Now: since the single payer system only focuses on the treatments and patients that produce a maximum of certain—or highly probable—QALYs, it can look as though the system is very efficient. In plain English: if we only cure very ill patients who will live for a long time afterward, and don't care about those who are either on the brink of dying, or only vaguely ill, or who may become ill soon—then it will look like we have gotten a lot of health care for little money.

In a free market system there is no room for a utilitarian dictator. There may be utilitarian-based decisions, but we do not have to subject our health needs to one single utilitarian regime. On the other hand, we can choose to spend more of our money on preventive care if we want to. Such care does not produce certain, or highly probable, QALYs, but the patient's experience is that his life has improved. And at the end of the day, that is all that matters.

Let me offer a personal experience to illustrate this point. My son had a mold that his mother and I were concerned about. At that time we lived in Denmark, which has one of the better working socialized health systems. I asked our family doctor to refer us to a dermatologist for evaluation. The dermatologist told me that: a) the mold was not atypical, i.e., would never become a seat of melanoma; and, b) even if it was atypical, they would not remove it until my son actually developed melanoma.

Upon moving to the United States a year later, I asked a dermatologist to evaluate the same mold. The answer: it should be removed because it was probably atypical. After surgery, the lab report confirmed that the mold was indeed atypical and could have developed melanoma many years into the future.

The Danish dermatologist barely glanced at the mold, and his reason was simple: even if it was atypical they would not have removed it anyway. The probability that removing the mold would save my son from a deadly cancer was simply not high enough.

As a parent, I am of course infinitely grateful for the recommendation by the American doctor that the mold be removed. I now know that my son is at less risk of developing a dangerous form of cancer. But according to the books of the single payer system, the utilitarian dictator would have denied me the right to have my son treated preventively. By those books, the surgery that my son underwent was unproductive. It has not cured a condition, only prevented a possible one. And since we will never know if the money was "wasted" or "well spent", the money should have been spent on something else.

Common sense says, of course, that the money that my son's surgery cost was indeed well spent. It improved our quality of life *as we see it*.

What makes the utilitarian dictator a dictator is the fact that single payer systems must emphasize cost containment—and that the decision to contain costs is made by one single body: the government health bureaucracy. They need to centralize their decision process to such a degree that individuals are eradicated and all that remains are abstract utility functions, QALYs and probabilities. Individual patients cannot have a say in what health care is offered and what is not offered. They just have to cope with whatever decisions the utilitarian dictator makes.

It is well known that American health care emphasizes preventive care much more than European systems do. This makes our health system look less efficient through a utilitarian prism.

The question, of course, is where would you like to be a patient?

Here is a blunt but accurate way of illustrating what the utilitarian dictator actually would do to our health care system (if we let him in):

1. since we want to keep costs down, we have to maximize the QALYs we produce with a given budget;

2. in order to maximize QALYs, we will only treat the really sick, because then we know that we will make an immediate, measurable difference;

3. therefore, we are going to discourage you from seeing a doctor until you are really sick.

By prioritizing cost containment over the freedom of health consumers (current and future patients) the single payer health system says that patients have to stand back when the state needs to balance its budget and keep costs down.

If we trust our politicians and health bureaucrats enough to believe that they will always decide in our favor, then sure—let us create a single payer health system. Let us submit our health needs to the decisions and rulings of a utilitarian dictator.

But if we are in any doubt; if we suspect that our politicians and bureaucrats may choose to let us, or someone we love, suffer in the name of cost containment; if we would rather maintain control over our health care, especially in critical life-or-death decisions; then we should get off the train to health care socialism right now.

Instead, we should make a serious effort to improve the free-market based system we have.

SO WHAT IS THE TAX BILL FOR SOCIALIZED HEALTH?

It is possible that our legislators will give us single payer health insurance despite all its agonizing downsides. I certainly hope not, but there is a tendency among those who want a single payer system to overlook the arguments we have discussed thus far.

Another suggestion that is often heard is that the government could run health care cheaper than the private sector. This claim obviously contradicts what we said about the inefficiencies of government-run health insurance. It also contradicts evidence that we will get to later, which shows the significant tax bills that come with single payer systems.

At times, I get the impression that some politicians—not all, and certainly not a majority, but a disturbingly large minority—hope that voters will be ignorant enough not to question the credibility of their proposals.

We, the public, on the other hand, assume that our elected officials will not try to deceive us. Unfortunately, the bigger government gets, the more it becomes a magnet for people who seek power more than anything else.

To make sure we can identify them and single them out, we need to educate ourselves. This is especially important when it comes to big and centennially important issues like health care reform. Learning more is the best way for us to take back control over our government and make sure it does not mess up our lives or waste our hard earned money.

A key to becoming more informed citizens is learning how to find, read and use statistical information. This chapter is a guide to how we can do that. It is a dense chapter, and if you are not used to working with numbers in this way, please take your time. It is worth it. If you learn to read and analyze basic statistical information, you will be able to outsmart most of your elected officials. (Yes, it's true!) You will be in a power position vs. those who want your vote.

This chapter is a guide to who you can find answers to the two most basic questions in the discussion about single payer health insurance:

1. How much money is spent on health care each year in a state, and how much of that is paid by taxpayers?

2. How much would it cost taxpayers, in a socialized health system, to give every resident the same health care as the average family gets today?

Let us use California as a real world example.

It takes only a few clicks and a tiny bit of addition and subtraction to get the answer to the first question. We start out with finding data on health care spending from the website of the U.S. Department of Health and Human Services. Their Center for Medicare and Medicaid Services has an excellent database:

http://www.cms.hhs.gov/NationalHealthExpendData/

Under the headline "National health expenditure data" in the upper left corner, we click on the word "state". That leads us to a new web page called "Health expenditures by state". Scrolling down a bit we find "Downloads".

Now we have to be careful so we get the right set of data. We are looking for "Health expenditures by state of provider: State-specific tables, 1980–2004"—or a later year than 2004, as updates come in.

This PDF file is 312 pages long. But we should not be deterred by its mere size. Once we know how to read this document, we have come a long way toward mastering the numbers and facts of universal health care.

The document's title is "Personal Health Care Expenditures (PHCE): All Persons". In the left margin is a list of all states. We click on our state—California, in this case—and get data for all personal health care expenditures in California from 1980 to 2004 (or later) spread out over two pages.

Before we start looking at the numbers, we have to understand one thing about PHCE. This is not all health spending that goes on in our country. There is also something called "Public health care spending" that comes on top of PHCE. When we add public and private health care spending together we get "National Health Expenditures", NHE.

So why are we not looking at NHE? It has to do with what single payer health care would be paying for. It does not bother with public health spending—it is about personal health care expenditures only. This includes the health care we get through our private, employer based insurance. It also accounts for health care paid for via Medicaid and Medicare, plus, of course, whatever we pay for out of pocket.

Public health spending, on the other hand, is the sum total of various health education projects that the federal, state and local governments have. These projects are often information campaigns. Some are temporary, others are permanent. They can be about how to avoid AIDS, how to keep teenage pregnancies down or how to quit smoking.

We the taxpayers are already paying for public health projects. So what really matters to us is how much it will cost to have a single payer universal health care program that covers all our personal health care expenditures.

Going back to our document over PHCE in California, we find a list of itemized spending in the far left column. The top category is, of course, the sum total of PHCE in the state each year, in millions of dollars. As the first column of numbers reveals, in 1980 California PHCE was $26,481 million. In simpler numbers: $26.5 billion.

Below the sum total are all the items—kinds—of spending that make up personal health care expenditures. The largest item in 1980 was "Hospital Care" with $11.6 billion (or "bn").

Below all the items that add up to personal health care, we have "Sources of funding (millions of dollars)". This headline is a little bit deceptive. It gives us the impression that we are going to learn about all the sources of health care funding. But only two sources are reported: Medicare and Medicaid. All private sources (such as employer based insurance, individual insurance purchases and out of pocket payments) have been left out. Of course, it is easy to figure out how much we actually spend through private funding:

Personal health care   - Medicare   - Medicaid   = <u>*Private health care expenditures*</u>

For our particular example, California in 1980, this translates into the following numbers:

Personal health care   - Medicare   - Medicaid   = <u>*Private health care expenditures*</u>

$26.5bn   - $4.2bn   - $3.0bn   = <u>$19.3 billion</u>

This seems so simple, almost trivial. But *we have already found an important piece of information* in our quest for the cost of a single payer system. We know how much private citizens in California are spending on health care—the $19.3 billion. This amount must of course be paid by taxes under a single payer system.

In addition, California will obviously also finance Medicare and Medicaid with taxes.

In order words, in answer to our first question—"How much money is spent on health care each year in a state, and how much of that is paid by taxpayers?"—we have found that:

- in California in 1980 the universal health program would have had to cover $26.5 billion in personal health spending;

- taxpayers already pay for $7.2 billion worth of Medicare and Medicaid. Therefore:

- under a single payer system, Californians would have had to pay at least $19.3 billion more in taxes back in 1980.

Let us now fast forward from 1980 to 2004. At the bottom of the screen is a small window with the page number, telling us that we are on page 31 of 312 pages total. Right next to it is an arrow. By clicking on it we move to page 32, which continues the same data series as we have just been looking at. We now have California's PHCE all the way up through 2004.

The top row tells us that Californians spent $169.1 billion on health care in 2004.

We subtract Medicare and Medicaid again:

Personal health care	- Medicare	- Medicaid	= Private health care expenditures
$169.1bn	- $32.2bn	- $28.8bn	= $108.1 billion

So with a single payer system, California taxpayers would have to pay $108.1 billion just to cover what they now are paying for through private insurance and out of pocket.

The final bill, though, is going to be higher. Since California wants a single payer system we add the Medicare costs. As we saw above, Medicare in California costs $32.2 billion. We also have to let the state pay all of the $28.8 billion Medicaid bill. Since states pay approximately 41 percent of Medicaid, we add 28.8 x 0.6 = $17.3 billion.

End result: a single payer system would increase the tax burden on California's taxpayers by $157.6 billion.

How much is this per taxpayer? To answer that, we must find some population data for California.

A good place to go for that information is the U.S. Census Bureau, which publishes detailed and interesting data on population and health coverage. (Yes, *interesting*!) Taxpayers are usually of working age, meaning 18–64 years old. Let us therefore identify that group.

We can do this by going to a web page on the Census website that will be of use to us both now and later on:

http://www.census.gov/hhes/www/hlthins/hlthins.html

In the middle of the screen we now have two yellow frames. The upper frame is called "Latest Health Insurance Data" and the lower frame is called "More Health Insurance Data". That is the one we are interested in. It has four links. We click on the third one, "Historical Health Insurance Tables".

This takes us to a page with links to nine different tables, called HI-1, HI-2, etc. up to HI-9. Each of these tables gives us a different perspective on health insurance coverage over the past 20 years. Since we are looking for data on state level coverage and—not to forget—population, we will focus on tables HI-4, HI-5 and HI-6.

First we click on table HI-6 and retrieve "Health Insurance Coverage Status and Type of Coverage by State—People Under 65: 1987 to 2005". The first table that we see is for the United States as a whole. We are looking for information on California, but before we scroll down to find it, let us just briefly get acquainted with how this table works.

The first column displays the calendar year (2005). The second one gives "all people", or the total number of Americans aged 0–64. That was 258.3 million in 2005. (Please note that the numbers are in thousands—so "258,330" is really "258,330 thousand" ...) The next column reveals the total number of people who were uninsured at any point in time during 2005 (46.1 million).

We then have a so called standard error number (321 in this case) which tells us that the Census data are estimates, not an exact counts. An exact count would have a standard error of zero.

After that we get the percent of uninsured, followed by another standard error and then the number of people who have private or tax paid public health insurance.

Let us stop here. We will explore the rest of the health coverage data later, but at this point it is more important that we retrieve the information we need for California. So we scroll down the web page until we find California. We then notice that in 2005 there were 32.1 million Californians aged 0–64.

To get the working age Californians out of that group, we obviously need to subtract children. To find that number we return to the page with the nine "HI" tables. We click on "HI-5" which gives us the same information as HI-6, but for children under 18 years of age.

This table has the same layout as the previous one, so we simply repeat the same procedure as before. We find that there were 9.7 million children in California in 2005. Subtracting these kids from the group aged 0–64 gives us the number of Californians of working age, 18–64.

That number is 22.4 million.

Now we are ready to find out how much a single payer health insurance system in California would cost each taxpayer. As we saw above, the total net cost to California taxpayers for a single payer system is going to be $157.6 billion. Divided up among 22.4 million working age Californians, we get $7,036 per year, per person.

For a family with two working parents, that means $14,072 per year.

This is, again, just to pay for exactly the health care that is provided today. We have not expanded coverage to the uninsured, nor have we increased or decreased health care quality.

We also have not accounted for the 12 percent expected efficiency losses in government run health care, as we discussed them earlier.

These are facts that we take into consideration when we answer the second question: "How much would it cost taxpayers, in a socialized health system, to give every resident the same health care as the average family gets today?"

The answer to this question is obviously not the same as the answer to the first question. To assure that we are providing health insurance for everybody we also have to count the uninsured.

In other words: we have to take the sum total of today's health care spending and spread it out so that it also covers the uninsured. In order to do this, let us go back to this web page:

http://www.census.gov/hhes/www/hlthins/hlthins.html

Once again, we click on "Historical Health Insurance Tables" and get the screen with the nine HI tables.

Last time we identified a number for the uninsured, it was from the table with people age 0–64. This time we need to find the number for all the uninsured in California. To do that we open table HI-4: "Health Insurance Coverage Status and Type of Coverage by State—All Persons".

Once again, we scroll down to California and find that in 2005 there were 6.9 million uninsured in California.

The uninsured are not entirely without health care. They get a fair amount of it for free. Estimates of how much they get vary a great deal, but a reasonable assumption is that they consume about half as much health care as those who are uninsured.

We therefore divide the uninsured population in half and add that number to the number of insured Californians.

Copy that? Since the 6.96 million uninsured are already consuming half of the health care they would do if they were fully insured, we simply assume that every other uninsured person gets all the health care they need, and every other gets nothing. Then we add those who get nothing and ignore those who "get" health care.

That gives us a total of 32.4 million health consumers.

We split the $169.1 billion among them and get a per capita health spending of $5,219.

This is the per capita health spending when every uninsured person gets the same amount of health care as the insured do. Without coverage for the uninsured, per capita health spending is $5,843. Covering the uninsured therefore reduces access to health care for the rest of the Californians by almost eleven percent.

While this sounds abstract, it means, in practice, that your doctor will no longer be able to spend a full hour examining you, but has to let you go after 53 minutes. You may have to wait longer than you are used to, in order to see him.

Not much of a hassle, especially since it is a good thing to cover the uninsured. The problem is—as we know by now—that single payer systems cost so much more than that. There are better ways to help the uninsured, as we will discuss in the Way Forward chapter.

But what would it cost if we wanted to avoid that eleven percent loss? Well, to find out we simply do the operation "backwards":

- the $5,843 is what each Californian wants to consume in health care;
- we need to find out how much this amounts to, in total;
- then we need to divide that up among the taxpayers.

If we give each Californian—including the uninsured—$5,843 worth of health care per year, we end up with a total bill of $209.8 billion. We subtract what the state is paying for Medicaid today, i.e., $11.5 billion. That leaves $198.3 billion to be sliced up among 22.4 million taxpayers.

The end result? $8,853 per taxpayer per year. Or <u>$17,706 for a family with two working parents</u>.

That is how much the health care tax alone would cost an average family.

A lot of money, of course. In fact, it is 27 percent more than we estimated without the uninsured.

To conclude this exercise, let us compare this number to the taxes that Californians are already paying. To find numbers on the current tax burden on California families, we go to another excellent website, namely the Bureau of Economic Analysis. The BEA is a federal agency that produces some of the best economic statistics in the world. They have excellent data on personal income, i.e., how much we earn.

For our needs, the best page on their website is:

<u>http://bea.gov/bea/regional/spi/</u>

The title of this page is "Annual State Personal Income". We can use it to get almost any information we want on personal income at the state level.

In three simple steps we can quickly retrieve the numbers that we need.

1. we select the last option on the list, "SA 50—Personal Income Taxes".

2. we choose the first option, "SA-50 Current Series (1958–2005)".

3. we click on California and the year 2005.

Then we click "Display". If you are well acquainted with Excel and CSV files, the "Download" option is a good one. If not, the "Display" option works well.

We now get a table with three columns: "code", "item" and "2005". Each code is attached to an item, obviously, and can be used to compare one particular item across all states in the country. We are not going to do that here, but it is a nice feature that we can play around with and learn a thing or two about our own state.

We stay focused on two items: personal income and personal taxes. Personal income is the first item. Our table tells us that in 2005 the sum total of all personal income, earned by all Californians together, was $1.3 trillion. Please note that the amount for personal income that the table reports, "$1,332,918,864", is actually *thousands of dollars*. We therefore have to add three zeros at the end so that the sum total of personal income in California reads: $1,332,918,864,000. Or $1.3 trillion.

In a moment we are going to divide this amount by the number of working age Californians.[32] But before we do that we need to find out what taxes Californians pay out of their personal income today—without any taxes to pay for a single payer system.

We therefore go to the next item under "Personal income", which is "Personal current taxes". It tells us that Californians paid $176.3 billion in personal taxes in 2005.

The bottom two thirds of the table give us a break-down of these taxes:

- $128.2 billion goes to the federal government,

- $45.8 billion goes to the state government, and

- $2.3 billion are local taxes.

Before we add the cost of the single payer health system on to our numbers, we first need to break these numbers down to our two-income family, which pays, per year …

- $11,446 in federal taxes, and

- $4,089 in state taxes.

This, plus the pocket change that goes to local governments, adds up to $15,741 per year, per family.

Enter the single payer health insurance system.

As we saw earlier, that system would come to cost the same family $17,706 per year in health care taxes. On top of all the other taxes.

In other words: if California's SB-840 single payer bill would become the law of the land, it would increase the tax burden on an average two-income California family by 112 percent.

Now that we know how to estimate the costs of single payer systems, let us look at some states where state legislators have proposed such systems. The list of states is not complete—it keeps growing almost by the day—and I have selected these states on two grounds only: the bills that have been proposed there are either comprehensive enough to be a credible proposal, or have some individual characteristic that made them particularly interesting at the time of publication of this book.

STATE-LEVEL SINGLE PAYER BILLS

If the federal government does nothing about health reform in 2008, the states will. There is a strong push for single payer systems at the state level. To show what this means in practice, in this chapter I go through a dozen examples of single-payer, universal health insurance bills at the state level. It is not a complete account of all the bills out there, but it samples the most elaborate proposals and offers insight both into the variety of bills out there and into one of their major weaknesses: they come with no estimates of how much they will cost taxpayers. (The other major weakness is that they do not even mention the serious health care rationing problems in Europe and Canada.)

The cost estimates are based on the premise that each state wants to create a single payer system. That is not the case with all the bills discussed, at least not explicitly. Some of the implicitly assume a single payer system, others—such as the Illinois bill—are for children and designed so that they can easily be expanded to cover all residents of the state. In those cases I report the numbers for both the "kids only" version and a hypothetical "all residents" version.

It is revealing to see how much the state-level single payer systems would cost taxpayers. In Missouri, e.g., state taxes would practically triple. In Connecticut, they would "only" double.

Equally revealing is the cost for a national single payer system. To run that system today, the federal government would have to raise taxes by $1.6 trillion. Today the federal government's spending is about $2.9 trillion. So it would essentially increase the federal government's size by 55 percent.

It deserves to be pointed out that some of the states discussed here already have universal health coverage, such as Maine and Vermont. But a state with universal health coverage does not necessarily have—universal health coverage. The only way to actually achieve universal coverage is to have a single payer system. So long as it is the private citizen's responsibility to pay for health insurance, there will be those among us who either choose not to buy insurance or who cannot afford it.

This is why I discuss single payer systems in Maine and Vermont, and not just universal coverage.

Single payer systems will cost us a lot of money not just by raising our taxes. They will also drain our health care systems of resources because they have a weaker output efficiency. As we noted before, this output efficiency loss is about 12 percent. I take this loss into account as I estimate what the individual state plans would actually cost taxpayers.

A word of caution before we move on to the state bills. The estimates of how much more taxes a two-income family would have to pay are not meant to be precise calculations. Such calculations would take long, and quite frankly rather tedious, discussions of our tax system. Instead, consider these tax cost estimates an indication of how much the average family might have to pay. If you make more than the average household, you will have to pay more. If you make less, you will—hopefully—have to pay less.

Here is a summary of what single payer systems would cost in the states studied (2004 numbers are used to assure full access to all relevant data):

UNITED STATES

Total estimated cost to taxpayers (2004):	**$1.6 trillion**
Health care income tax, average two-income family:	**$17,222** per year

CALIFORNIA

Total estimated cost to taxpayers (2004):	**$193.8 billion**
Health care income tax, average two-income family:	**$17,328** per year

CONNECTICUT

Total estimated cost to taxpayers (2004):	**$24.3 billion**
Health care income tax, average two-income family:	**$22,124** per year

HAWAII

Total estimated cost to taxpayers (2004):	**$7.06 billion**
Health care income tax, average two-income family:	**$18,020** per year

ILLINOIS

Total estimated cost to taxpayers (2004):	**$73.6 billion**
Health care income tax, average two-income family:	**$18,868** per year

KANSAS

Total estimated cost to taxpayers (2004):   **$15.9 billion**

Health care income tax, average two-income family: **$19,166** per year

MAINE

Total estimated cost to taxpayers (2004):   **$8.5 billion**

Health care income tax, average two-income family: **$20,472** per year

MARYLAND

Total estimated cost to taxpayers (2004):   **$34.5 billion**

Health care income tax, average two-income family: **$19,632** per year

MISSOURI

Total estimated cost to taxpayers (2004):   **$36.4 billion**

Health care income tax, average two-income family: **$18,892** per year

NEW YORK

Total estimated cost to taxpayers (2004):   **$134.8 billion**

Health care income tax, average two-income family: **$22,512** per year

OHIO

Total estimated cost to taxpayers (2004):   **$77.4 billion**

Health care income tax, average two-income family: **$21,801** per year

VERMONT

Total estimated cost to taxpayers (2004):   **$3.9 billion**

Health care income tax, average two-income family: **$19,548** per year

WISCONSIN

Total estimated cost to taxpayers (2004):   **$34.8 billion**

Health care income tax, average two-income family: **$22,948** per year

UNITED STATES

Total estimated cost to taxpayers (2004): **$1.6 trillion**

Health care income tax, average two-income family: **$17,222** per year

Total tax bill incl. current taxes (two-income family): **$28,754** per year[33]

As we have already seen, the Democratic party is full of advocates for universal, single payer health insurance. The one piece that is missing, though, is their assessment of how much their plans would cost taxpayers. The following is an example of how we can determine that cost.

COST OF A SINGLE PAYER SYSTEM TO AMERICA'S TAXPAYERS

In 2004, we the people of the United States of America spent $1.6 trillion on personal health care. Let us extend full coverage to all the 45.8 million uninsured nationwide. We assume that they are already getting half of the health care they need under the current system, so full coverage for them adds $251.8 billion to the total spending.

We now have $1.85 trillion worth of personal health expenditures that our Federal government will have to cover.

Of course, it would not have to come up with all of that. It is already paying 59 percent of all Medicaid expenses in the country, plus Medicare. We subtract these items from the aforementioned $1.85 trillion, and end up with $1.4 trillion. We then adjust the amount for the expected 12 percent efficiency loss from socializing health care. The end result: $1.56 trillion that the Federal government will have to raise in the form of new taxes.

The most logical source of those taxes is personal income. To estimate how much more of our personal income the Federal government would claim, let us first define the group of taxpayers that would be burdened with this tax.

Almost everybody who earns personal income is from 18 to 64 years old. There are 182.1 million working age Americans. If we split the $1.56 trillion among them, they each have to pay a health care tax of $8,611 per year.

For an average family with two working parents this amounts to $17,222 per year in health care taxes alone.

We then have to add this to all the other taxes they are paying.

In total, federal, state and local taxes on personal income in the United States in 2004 was $1.05 trillion, or $11,532 per month per two-income family.

We now add the health care tax to this amount. Our sum total: **$28,754** per year for a family with two working parents.

CALIFORNIA

Bill name	California Health Insurance Reliability Act
Bill number	SB-840
Principal sponsor	Senator Sheila Kuehl, D-Santa Monica
Reform type	Universal, single payer health care

Total estimated cost to taxpayers (2004): **$193.8 billion**

Health care income tax, average two-income family: **$17,328** per year

Total tax bill incl. current taxes (two-income family): **$30,876** per year

When Governor Schwarzenegger vetoed SB-840, he did it with two motivations: it was not the right solution to California's health care crisis, and it would require "billions" in new taxes. The first motive is hardly to be taken seriously, as the governor did not offer his own solution. The second motive, though, is important and shows that Governor Schwarzenegger has a good understanding of the economic importance of free markets and limited government.

The governor's office has not produced any detailed assessments of the cost of SB-840. It is hardly the governor's responsibility, since he is not the author of the universal health proposal. Nevertheless, it would be helpful to the governor's own attempts at reforming California's health insurance system if he could present voters with the truly horrifying tax costs behind SB-840.

Below is an estimate of that cost. If anything, it verifies the governor's fears that a universal, single payer health insurance system would deal a terrible tax blow to the Californian economy.

COST OF THE PLAN

In 2004, the people of California spent $169.1 billion on personal health care. Then we extend full coverage to all the 6.7 million uninsured in California. We assume that they are already getting half of the health care they need under the current system, so full coverage for them adds $15.8 billion to the total spending.

We now have $184.9 billion worth of personal health expenditures that the state of California will have to cover.

Of course, the state would not have to come up with all of that. It is already paying 41 percent of the $28.8 billion worth of Medicaid spending in the state.

We therefore subtract $11.8 billion from total personal health expenditures. This leaves us with $173 billion. We then adjust for the expected 12 percent efficiency loss and we have $193.8 billion that the state has to raise through new state income taxes.

Almost everybody who earns personal income is from 18 to 64 years old. There are 22.4 million working age Californians. If we split the $193.8 billion among them, they each have to pay a health care tax of $8,664 per year.

For an average family with two working parents this amounts to $17,328 per year in health care taxes alone.

We then have to add this to all the other taxes they are paying.

In total, federal, state and local taxes on personal income in California in 2004 was $151.5 billion, or $13,548 per month per two-income family.

We now add the health care tax to this amount. Our sum total: **$30,876** per year for a family with two working parents.

CONNECTICUT

Bill name	AN ACT CONCERNING HEALTH CARE SECURITY
Bill number	Senate Bill 482
Introduced by	Human Services Committee
Reform type	Universal, single payer health care

Total estimated cost to taxpayers (2004): **$24.3 billion**

Health care income tax, average two-income family: **$22,124** per year

Total tax bill incl. current taxes (two-income family): **$43,463** per year

This bill wants to monopolize health care in the hands of the state government. The state would "set or establish methods for setting rates, fees and prices for the Connecticut health care system and reviewing the sufficiency of such rates, fees and prices".[34]

This bill is only the latest example of a state level push for socialized health in Connecticut. In January 2005 Representative Geragosian introduced a brief bill, HB 6303, that also sought universal single payer health care. That bill was referred to the state legislature's Joint Committee on Public Health and scheduled for a public hearing on March 14, 2005. It was essentially a renewed attempt to introduce universal, single payer health insurance in Connecticut after State House Bill 5872 failed in 2001. Representative John C Geragosian was one of the sponsors behind that bill; he is the sole sponsor of Bill 6003.

Connecticut state legislators who want socialized health are apparently taking a step by step approach to that goal. On September 29, 2006 State Senator Donald J DeFronzo announced that he and a group of other legislators had achieved $2.5 million in funding for a new health center for low income families in New Britain. The news release about the funding quotes Representative John C Geragosian as saying:

"I'm proud of the facility in New Britain, and I think they *[similar centers]* are part of our plan to achieve *universal health care* for everyone."[35]

Nowhere in his House Bill 6303, or supporting documents, does Representative Geragosian make any effort to estimate how much his bill would cost taxpayers.

The push for universal, single payer health insurance in Connecticut is backed by the Connecticut Coalition for Universal Health Care. On its website[36] the Coalition presents data on how rapidly health care expenditures are rising in America. They use these numbers as indirect support for their universal health argument. However, the Coalition also fails to mention that the very expenditures that they are relaying would be paid entirely by working families in a universal health system.

Either that, or working families will have to face serious health care rationing, with Canadian, if not Swedish waiting lists to see a doctor.

COST OF THE PLAN

In 2004, the people of Connecticut spent $22 billion on personal health care. Then we extend full coverage to all the 407,000 uninsured in Connecticut. We assume that they are already getting half of the health care they need under the current system, so full coverage for them adds $1.3 billion to the total spending.

We now have $23.3 billion worth of personal health expenditures that the state of Connecticut will have to cover.

Of course, the state would not have to come up with all of the $23.3 billion. It is already paying 41 percent of the $3.8 billion worth of Medicaid spending in the state. To find out what the state genuinely has to fund, we therefore subtract $1.6 billion from total personal health expenditures. This leaves us with $21.7 billion. Adjusting for the expected 12 percent efficiency loss, we end up with 24.3 billion that the state must collect through state income taxes.

Almost everybody who earns personal income is from 18 to 64 years old. There are 2,195,000 working age people in Connecticut. If we split the $24.3 billion among them, they each have to pay a health care tax of $11,068 per year.

For an average family with two working parents this amounts to $22,124 per year in health care taxes alone.

We then have to add this to all the other taxes they are paying.

In total, federal, state and local taxes on personal income in Connecticut in 2004 was $23.4 billion, or $21,342 per working age resident.

We now add the health care tax to this amount. Our sum total: **$43,463** for a family with two working parents.

HAWAII

Bill number	Several different
Reform type	Universal single payer health care

Total estimated cost to taxpayers (2004): **$7.06 billion**

Health care income tax, average two-income family: **$18,020** per year

Total tax bill incl. current taxes (two-income family): **$29,110** per year

COST OF THE PLAN

In 2004, the people of Hawaii spent $6.3 billion on personal health care. In compliance with a universal, single payer health system we extend full coverage to all the 120,000 uninsured in Hawaii. We assume that they are already getting half of the health care they need under the current system, so full coverage for them adds $301 million to the total spending.

We now have $6.6 billion worth of personal health expenditures that the state of Hawaii will have to cover.

Of course, the state would not have to come up with all of that. It is already paying 41 percent of the Medicaid spending in the state. We therefore subtract $339 million from total personal health expenditures. This leaves us with $6.3 billion. Adjusting for the expected 12 percent efficiency loss under a single payer system, we end up with a need to fund $7.06 billion through state income taxes.

Almost everybody who earns personal income is from 18 to 64 years old. There are 782,000 working age residents in Hawaii. If we split the $7.06 billion among them, they each have to pay <u>a health care tax of $9,010</u> per year.

For an average family with two working parents this amounts to <u>$18,020 per year in health care taxes alone</u>.

We then add this to all the other taxes they are paying.

In total, federal, state and local taxes on personal income in Hawaii in 2004 was $4.3 billion, or $11,090 per year per two-income family.

We now add the health care tax to this amount. Our sum total: **$29,110** per year for a family with two working parents.

ILLINOIS

Bill name	Covering ALL KIDS Insurance Act; Amendment
Bill number	House Bill 806
Principal sponsor	Senator Emil Jones Jr.
Reform type	Universal health coverage for children

For this particular bill:

Total estimated cost to taxpayers (**2003**): **$7.1 billion**

Health care income tax, average two-income family: **$1,800** per year

Total tax bill incl. current taxes (two-income family): **$13,728** per year

For universal health care (not part of this bill):

Total estimated cost to taxpayers (**2004**): **$73.6 billion**

Health care income tax, average two-income family: **$18,868** per year

Total tax bill incl. current taxes (two-income family): **$31,174** per year

This plan is for children only. It is relatively easy to estimate its direct costs, but because it only covers children there will be indirect effects that raise the cost of it significantly. These indirect effects come in the form of more adults without insurance.

Children are relatively cheap to insure, which means that they are more profitable to insurers than adults. With children in the risk pool insurers can balance the high risk adults against low risk kids.

This means that there will be little or no drop in insurance premiums if only parents buy them. As an indication of this, consider a typical private health insurance in Illinois with 20 percent co-insurance, $25 per visit to a medical office and $2,500 deductible.[37] This policy costs virtually the same—about $450 per month—if a couple applies with or without children. The only significant change is a drop in the deductible to $1,000.

There is of course a wide variety in the cost, design and coverage of insurance plans, but the variety is more due to the design of individual plans than whether or not children are enrolled. Children constitute a relatively low risk to health insurance providers, and once they are removed from the risk pool (i.e., once they are on tax paid insurance) the insurance providers are left with a higher risk clientele.

While parents will probably face the same health insurance premiums once their kids are on tax paid insurance, they will also have to pay higher taxes. As shown below, the taxes needed to pay health insurance for all Illinois kids will definitely be noticed in most family budgets.

COST OF THE PLAN TO INSURE ALL CHILDREN

To estimate the direct direct cost of Illinois House Bill 806 we are going to use data from 2003 published by the Center for Medicaid and Medicare Services (an office within the U.S. Department of Health and Human Services). That year, Medicaid spending on children in Illinois was $1.6 billion. There were 663,000 children on Medicaid, which means $2,413 per child.

Today the Federal government pays most of that cost, but under a universal, single payer plan for kids in Illinois, the state would be responsible for the entire cost for every child. And that is *every* child in the state, not just those on Medicaid.

In 2003 there were 3,210,000 children in Illinois. How much would it cost to cover them all?

First, the state will have to replace federal funds for the kids who are currently on Medicaid. That is $1 billion. Then the state has to pay $2,413 for each one of the remaining 2.5 million kids who are currently either on private insurance or uninsured. Cost: $6.1 billion.

This tallies up to $7.1 billion. That is the total cost for expanding tax paid health insurance to all kids in Illinois.

Where would the state of Illinois find that kind of money? One way or the other it will be up to regular middle class taxpayers to pay for it. There just aren't enough rich folks around.

To put some proportions on the cost, the state would have to *practically double its income taxes.*

WHAT WOULD A SINGLE PAYER, UNIVERSAL HEALTH SYSTEM COST?

If Illinois, some time in the future, were to move to a universal, single payer system, the costs would obviously be much higher than for a system that only covers children.

In 2004, the people of Illinois spent $65.2 billion on personal health care. Then we extend full coverage to all the 1.8 million uninsured in Illinois. We assume that they are already getting half of the health care they need under the current system, so full coverage for them adds $4.6 billion to the total spending.

We now have $69.8 billion worth of personal health expenditures that the state of Illinois will have to cover.

Of course, the state would not have to come up with all of that. It is already paying 41 percent of the $10.1 billion worth of Medicaid spending in the state. We therefore subtract $4.1 billion from total personal health expenditures. This leaves us with $65.7 billion. Adjusting for the expected 12 percent efficiency loss, we have to fund $73.6 billion through state income taxes.

Almost everybody who earns personal income is from 18 to 64 years old. There are 7.8 million working age residents in Illinois. If we split the $73.6 billion among them, they each have to pay a health care tax of $9,434 per year.

For an average family with two working parents this amounts to $18,868 per year in health care taxes alone.

We then have to add this to all the other taxes they are paying.

In total, federal, state and local taxes on personal income in Illinois in 2004 was $48 billion, or $12,306 per month per two-income family.

We now add the health care tax to this amount. Our sum total: **$31,174** per year for a family with two working parents.

KANSAS

Bill name	House Bill no. 2001
Principal sponsor	Representatives Swenson and Powers
Reform type	Universal single payer health care

Total estimated cost to taxpayers (2004): **$15.9 billion**

Health care income tax, average two-income family: **$19,166** per year

Total tax bill incl. current taxes (two-income family): **$29,014** per year

In 2004, the people of Kansas spent $14.1 billion on personal health care. In compliance with a universal, single payer health system we extend full coverage to all the 297,000 uninsured in Kansas. We assume that they are already getting half of the health care they need under the current system, so full coverage for them adds $784 million to the total spending.

We now have $14.9 billion worth of personal health expenditures that the state of Kansas will have to cover.

Of course, the state would not have to come up with all of that. It is already paying 41 percent of the Medicaid spending in the state. We therefore subtract $708 million from total personal health expenditures. This leaves us with $14.2 billion. Adjusting for the expected 12 percent efficiency loss, we need to fund $15.9 billion through state income taxes.

Almost everybody who earns personal income is from 18 to 64 years old. There are 1,658,000 working age residents in Kansas. If we split the $15.9 billion among them, they each have to pay <u>a health care tax of $9,583</u> per year.

For an average family with two working parents this amounts to <u>$19,166 per year in health care taxes alone</u>.

We then add this to all the other taxes they are paying.

In total, federal, state and local taxes on personal income in Kansas in 2004 was $8.2 billion, or $9,848 per year per two-income family.

We now add the health care tax to this amount. Our sum total: <u>**$29,014**</u> per year for a family with two working parents.

MAINE

Bill name   HP 106

Principal sponsor   Representative Joanne Twomey

Reform type   Universal single payer health care

Total estimated cost to taxpayers (2004): **$8.5 billion**

Health care income tax, average two-income family: **$20,472** per year

Total tax bill incl. current taxes (two-income family): **$29,998** per year

In 2004, the people of Maine spent $8 billion on personal health care. In compliance with a universal, single payer health system we extend full coverage to all the 130,000 uninsured in Maine. We assume that they are already getting half of the health care they need under the current system, so full coverage for them adds $401 million to the total spending.

We now have $8.4 billion worth of personal health expenditures that the state of Maine will have to cover.

Of course, the state would not have to come up with all of that. It is already paying 41 percent of the Medicaid spending in the state. We therefore subtract $820 million from total personal health expenditures. This leaves us with $7.6 billion. Adjusting for the expected 12 percent efficiency loss, we need to fund $8.5 billion through state income taxes.

Almost everybody who earns personal income is from 18 to 64 years old. There are 828,000 working age residents in Maine. If we split the $8.5 billion among them, they each have to pay <u>a health care tax of $10,236</u> per year.

For an average family with two working parents this amounts to <u>$20,472 per year in health care taxes alone</u>.

We then add this to all the other taxes they are paying.

In total, federal, state and local taxes on personal income in Maine in 2004 were $3.9 billion, or $9,526 per year per two-income family.

We now add the health care tax to this amount. Our sum total: **$29,998** per year for a family with two working parents.

MARYLAND

Bill name	SB 727
Principal sponsor	Senator Pinsky
Reform type	Universal health insurance

Total estimated cost to taxpayers (2004): **$34.5 billion**

Health care income tax, average two-income family: **$19,632** per year

Total tax bill incl. current taxes (two-income family): **$35,932** per year

In 2004, the people of Maryland spent $30.4 billion on personal health care. In compliance with a universal, single payer health system we extend full coverage to all the 810,000 uninsured in Maryland. We assume that they are already getting half of the health care they need under the current system, so full coverage for them adds $2.2 billion to the total spending.

We now have $32.6 billion worth of personal health expenditures that the state of Maryland will have to cover.

Of course, the state would not have to come up with all of that. It is already paying 41 percent of the Medicaid spending in the state. We therefore subtract $1.8 billion from total personal health expenditures. This leaves us with $30.8 billion. Adjusting for the expected 12 percent efficiency loss, we need to fund $34.5 billion through state income taxes.

Almost everybody who earns personal income is from 18 to 64 years old. There are 3.5 million working age residents in Maryland. If we split the $34.5 billion among them, they each have to pay a health care tax of $9,816 per year.

For an average family with two working parents this amounts to $19,632 per year in health care taxes alone.

We then add this to all the other taxes they are paying.

In total, federal, state and local taxes on personal income in Maryland in 2004 was $28.7 billion, or $16,300 per year per two-income family.

We now add the health care tax to this amount. Our sum total: **$35,932** per year for a family with two working parents.

MISSOURI

Bill name	House Bill no. 80
Principal sponsor	Representative Bland
Reform type	Universal single payer health care

Total estimated cost to taxpayers (2004): **$36.4 billion**

Health care income tax, average two-income family: **$18,892** per year

Total tax bill incl. current taxes (two-income family): **$27,638** per year

In 2004, the people of Missouri spent $32.8 billion on personal health care. In compliance with a universal, single payer health system we extend full coverage to all the 707,000 uninsured in Missouri. We assume that they are already getting half of the health care they need under the current system, so full coverage for them adds $2.1 billion to the total spending.

We now have $34.9 billion worth of personal health expenditures that the state of Missouri will have to cover.

Of course, the state would not have to come up with all of that. It is already paying 41 percent of the Medicaid spending in the state. We therefore subtract $2.4 billion from total personal health expenditures. This leaves us with $32.5 billion. Adjusting for the expected 12 percent efficiency loss, we need to fund 36.4 billion through state income taxes.

Almost everybody who earns personal income is from 18 to 64 years old. There are 3.8 million working age residents in Missouri. If we split the $36.4 billion among them, they each have to pay a health care tax of $9,446 per year.

For an average family with two working parents this amounts to $18,892 per year in health care taxes alone.

We then add this to all the other taxes they are paying.

In total, federal, state and local taxes on personal income in Missouri in 2004 was $16.8 billion, or $8,746 per year per two-income family.

We now add the health care tax to this amount. Our sum total: **$27,638** per year for a family with two working parents.

NEW YORK

Bill name	A 07069
Principal sponsor	Assemblyman Colton
Reform type	Universal single payer health care

Total estimated cost to taxpayers (2004): **$134.8 billion**

Health care income tax, average two-income family: **$22,512** per year

Total tax bill incl. current taxes (two-income family): **$39,972** per year

In 2004, New Yorkers spent $127.9 billion on personal health care. In compliance with a universal, single payer health system we extend full coverage to all the 2.7 million uninsured in New York. We assume that they are already getting half of the health care they need under the current system, so full coverage for them adds $9.1 billion to the total spending.

We now have $137 billion worth of personal health expenditures that the state of New York will have to cover.

Of course, the state would not have to come up with all of that. It is already paying 41 percent of the Medicaid spending in the state. We therefore subtract $16.6 billion from total personal health expenditures. This leaves us with $120.4 billion. Adjusting for the expected 12 percent efficiency loss, we need to fund $134.8 through state income taxes.

Almost everybody who earns personal income is from 18 to 64 years old. There are 12 working age residents in New York. If we split the $120.4 billion among them, they each have to pay a health care tax of $11,256 per year.

For an average family with two working parents this amounts to $22,512 per year in health care taxes alone.

We then add this to all the other taxes they are paying.

In total, federal, state and local taxes on personal income in New York in 2004 was $104.5 billion, or $17,460 per year per two-income family.

We now add the health care tax to this amount. Our sum total: **$39,972** per year for a family with two working parents.

OHIO

Bill name	SB no. 263
Principal sponsor	Senators Hagan, Miller, Fedor, Brady
Reform type	Universal health insurance

Combined state-federal funding:

Total estimated cost to taxpayers (2004): **$55.0 billion**

Health care income tax, average two-income family: **$15,493** per year

Total tax bill incl. current taxes (two-income family): **$25,563** per year

State-only single payer model (not proposed in this bill):

Total estimated cost to taxpayers (2004): **$77.4 billion**

Health care income tax, average two-income family: **$21,801** per year

Total tax bill incl. current taxes (two-income family): **$32,871** per year

Technically, the Ohio model is not a single payer model in the traditional sense. It anticipates that the state will be receiving federal funds for Medicare and Medicaid, leaving it to the state to fund the rest. As the numbers above indicate, this makes a small difference to tax paying Ohioans. But the difference could become bigger: there is a chance that the federal government could decide to sponsor Ohio style plans, where funding is shared between the federal and state levels.

The Ohio plan is full of tempting promises of all the kinds of health care that will be provided to everyone, including "homeless and migrant workers". But the authors of the plan are also very well aware that their plan is going to cost a whole lot of money (although they apparently have not estimated the true cost of it). In Section 3922.09 of their bill they make clear that there will be an absolute cap on how much health care will cost. There will be a budget at the beginning of the fiscal year, and if health care ends up costing more than that, then they will exercise cost containment even if it means denying people health care:

The administrator of finance of the Ohio health care agency shall notify the Ohio health care board when the annual expenditures or anticipated future expenditures of the Ohio health care plan appear to be in excess of the revenues or anticipated revenues for the same period. The Ohio health care board shall implement appropriate cost control measures based on the notification.

If their efforts to ration health care are not strong enough, they will have to go to the state legislature and ask for more money:

The Ohio health care board shall seek a special appropriation for the Ohio health care fund if the cost control measures implemented do not reduce the Ohio health care plan's expenditures to an amount that may be covered by its revenue.

In other words: first the state's health bureaucrats will do everything they can to cut away health care for Ohio's families. Then, once quality has been deteriorated, waiting lists have skyrocketed and people are angry about how little they are getting for their tax dollars—then, the health bureaucrats will go to the legislators and ask for more of taxpayers' money to pay for the same deteriorated health care.

It is disturbing, quite frankly, to see this in a universal health insurance bill, because it means that the authors of that bill have not learned anything from the experiences of countries that already have universal health insurance. This is exactly what happens in those countries over and over again. The only outcome is deteriorating health care and higher taxes.

COST OF UNIVERSAL HEALTH INSURANCE IN OHIO

In 2004, Ohioans spent $65.4 billion on personal health care. In compliance with a universal, single payer health system we extend full coverage to all the 1.3 million uninsured in Ohio. We assume that they are already getting half of the health care they need under the current system, so full coverage for them adds $3.7 billion to the total spending.

We now have $69.1 billion worth of personal health expenditures that the state of Ohio will have to cover.

Of course, the state would not have to come up with all of that. Under the current bill, the state would still receive federal funds for Medicare and Medicaid. Today, federal funds pay 29 percent of Ohio's personal health expenditures. Let us assume that the universal health system in Ohio would still be funded up to that amount by federal money.

Since the Ohio system would be administered by one state bureaucracy, it will suffer from the same inefficiencies as any full single-payer system. Therefore, we adjust the $69.1 billion for the expected 12 percent efficiency loss. This gives us $77.4 billion. The Ohio bill expects the federal government to pay 29 percent of that, or $22.4 billion, or $2.4 billion more than before the efficiency loss.

Will the U.S. Congress merrily dole out the extra billions? Probably not, but let us assume that they do. We now split the state share of the whole cost among the 7.1 million working age Ohioans. They each end up having to pay a health care tax of $7,042 per year.

For an average family with two working parents this amounts to $15,493 per year in health care taxes alone.

Federal, state and local taxes on personal income in Ohio in 2004 was $39.3 billion, or $11,070 per year per two-income family.

We now add the health care tax to this amount. Our sum total: **$25,563** per year for a family with two working parents.

If Ohio would fund its universal health insurance system on its own, the health care tax would obviously be higher, as the numbers above indicate.

VERMONT

Bill name	H.0524
Principal sponsor	Representative Russell
Reform type	Universal health insurance

Total estimated cost to taxpayers (2004): **$3.9 billion**

Health care income tax, average two-income family: **$19,548** per year

Total tax bill incl. current taxes (two-income family): **$29,173** per year

If H.0524 would become the law of the land in Vermont, state taxpayers and health care consumers would be in trouble. The primary purpose of the bill is to contain costs:

> Health care costs have risen an average of 9–10 percent per year over the past 30–40 years, with the rate rising to 10–11 percent in more recent years. These figures are well above the Consumer Price Index and, moreover, exceed by far the state's capacity to pay for health care costs as measured against our gross state product and personal income. For example, between 1996 and 2002, health care spending in Vermont rose 63 percent, while personal income rose 41 percent and the gross state product rose 35 percent.

In other words, the idea is to tie the increase in health care spending to either personal income or gross state product. Under a universal, single payer system, the state of Vermont would impose health care rationing and dictate to the people of Vermont how much health care they can consume each year.

To understand what this means, let us assume that this bill had been enacted in 1990. We assume that the state allows health expenditures to grow with state GDP plus population change, just as in California's SB-840. Over the next 14 years, through 2004, the people of Vermont would lose a total of almost $1 billion worth of health care.

This loss does not even include the losses that the government itself causes, with its inevitable inefficiencies. We discussed these earlier (ref.) and noted that we can expect a loss of 8–12 percent of health care spending under the government. So let us factor in an eight percent efficiency loss.

Now things are getting a bit scary. Every year, on average, Vermonters would lose 11 percent in health care spending.

In 2004 alone Vermont's health care system would have lost $306 million dollars.

How much money is this, to a health care system like Vermont's? Well, let's crunch the numbers. In 2004 there were 42,000 people employed in the health sector in Vermont. The average annual cost to hire one of them is approximately $50,000. If we take $306 million out of health spending in Vermont, we end up having to **fire 6,100 health care workers.**

Another way of looking at it: taking $306 million out of Vermont's health care spending amounts to closing down some 400 health care establishments (such as physician's offices and specialist clinics) across the state.[38]

Obviously, this is not something that the universal health sponsors in Vermont have in mind. But it is exactly what they are going to have to do. This is what has happened in Scandinavia, which—like it or not—is the model that Vermont's health care socialists are glancing at. Small, rural hospitals, clinics and physician's offices are being closed in the name of cost containment. Patients have to travel far to wait to see a doctor at a major hospital. Women who are about to give birth can be forced to travel for an hour, or more, *even if they live in small cities.*

This is the grim, harsh reality of universal, single payer health care. When cost containment is made the highest priority—as it is in Vermont—the end result is always that bureaucrats and politicians take away what patients really need: doctors, nurses, dental care, prescription drug coverage, treatment with no waiting time …

THE COST OF SINGLE PAYER HEALTH INSURANCE IN VERMONT

In 2004, the people of Vermont spent $3.6 billion on personal health care. In compliance with a universal, single payer health system we extend full coverage to all the 69,000 uninsured in Vermont. We assume that they are already getting half of the health care they need under the current system, so full coverage for them adds $201 million to the total spending.

We now have $3.8 billion worth of personal health expenditures that the state of Vermont will have to cover.

Of course, the state would not have to come up with all of that. It is already paying 41 percent of the Medicaid spending in the state. We therefore subtract $312 million from total personal health expenditures. This leaves us with $3.5

billion. Adjusting for the expected 12 percent efficiency loss, we need to fund $3.9 billion through state income taxes.

Almost everybody who earns personal income is from 18 to 64 years old. There are 400,000 working age residents in Vermont. If we split the $3.9 billion among them, they each have to pay a health care tax of $9,774 per year.

For an average family with two working parents this amounts to $19,548 per year in health care taxes alone.

We then add this to all the other taxes they are paying.

In total, federal, state and local taxes on personal income in Vermont in 2004 was $1.9 billion, or $9,625 per year per two income family.

We now add the health care tax to this amount. Our sum total: **$29,173** per year for a family with two working parents.

WISCONSIN

Bill name	SB 388
Principal sponsor	Senators Miller, Carpenter, Erpenbach, Risser, Robson, Wirch
Reform type	Universal health insurance

Current bill with federal funds for Medicare and Medicaid:

Total estimated cost to taxpayers (2004): **$24.5 billion**

Health care income tax, average two-income family: **$14,420** per year

Total tax bill incl. current taxes (two-income family): **$25,575** per year

As a state-only single payer system (not proposed in this bill):

Total estimated cost to taxpayers (2004): **$34.8 billion**

Health care income tax, average two-income family: **$22,948** per year

Total tax bill incl. current taxes (two-income family): **$34,103** per year

The Wisconsin bill is unique among the universal health bills in this study: it comes with a "Fiscal Estimate"[39] that at least gives the impression of assessing the bill's cost. The problem is that the "fiscal estimate" does not really do what it sounds like it is doing. The sponsors of the bill have not been able to come up with even remotely credible numbers for what this plan would cost taxpayers. In fact, the state Executive Budget Finance office notes that the bill "does not appropriate funding to plan, implement or provide universal health care".[40] Instead, the bill wants a government Department of Public Health and Finance that will come up with a way to fund the whole plan—*after* the bill has been passed.

To further increase the threat of a massive tax hike to pay for the plan, the authors of the bill promise that the state will be the "payer of last resort" for health care. What this means, in plain English, is that private health plans no longer have to cover all that much, because the state will pick up the tab where they left off.

This is *an invitation to private employers to opt for the cheapest, thinnest health coverage possible* and then leave it up to the state to pay for most, if not all, of people's health care.

The bill's authors try to come across as prudent and thoughtful. They want to give the impression that they are looking at a limited coverage, not a sweeping universal system. Instead of granting everyone "comprehensive" coverage, the bill speaks of "reasonable medical services necessary to maintain health, enable diagnosis and provide treatment or rehabilitation for an injury, disability or disease". However, if this bill ever became law, the people of Wisconsin will soon find out that there is no upper end to how much health care the state will end up paying for.

To further conceal the risk of massive tax hikes, the bill assumes that the federal government will still pay for Medicare and most of Medicaid, and that private insurance will cover whatever is not included in the "reasonable health services" that the state pays for (perhaps those are "unreasonable" health services?). But the bill is already so generous that it would only take a minor adjustment to create a full fledged universal, single payer system. Here is what the bill means by reasonable health services—today already:

- Health services currently provided by existing, authorized health care facilities

- Preventive health care services, including well-child care, immunizations, screening, outreach and public health education

- Medical or surgical supplies and durable medical or surgical equipment, supplies and appliances, including—among many other things—eyeglasses

- A substantial coverage of prescription drugs

- Long term care services necessary for the physical, mental and emotional well-being, as well as social and personal needs of individuals with limited self-care capabilities

- Mental health including substance abuse

- Dental care

With all this paid for by the state, Wisconsin would have more generous tax paid health insurance than the Scandinavian countries. Over there, the government does not cover eyeglasses, and dental care is mostly or entirely private. Coverage for prescription drugs is also strictly limited.

The biggest problem is, of course, that the Wisconsin plan leaves so little to private insurance plans that it is basically pointless for an employer to offer any meaningful insurance to his employees. Once that happens, the system will quickly become a universal, single payer system.

THE COST OF SINGLE PAYER HEALTH INSURANCE IN WISCONSIN

In 2004, the people of Wisconsin spent $31.2 billion on personal health care. In compliance with a universal, single payer health system we extend full coverage to all the 566,000 uninsured in Wisconsin. We assume that they are already getting half of the health care they need under the current system, so full coverage for them adds $1.6 billion to the total spending.

We now have $32.8 billion worth of personal health expenditures. Of course, the state would not have to come up with all of that. It is already paying 41 per-cent of the Medicaid spending in the state. We therefore subtract $1.7 billion from total personal health expenditures. This leaves us with $31.1 billion. Adjusted for the expected 12 percent efficiency loss, we end up having to finance $34.8 billion through state income taxes.

Almost everybody who earns personal income is from 18 to 64 years old. There are 3.4 million working age residents in Wisconsin. If we split the $34.8 billion among them, they each have to pay a health care tax of $11,474 per year.

For an average family with two working parents this amounts to <u>$22,948 per year in health care taxes alone</u>.

We then add this to all the other taxes they are paying.

In total, federal, state and local taxes on personal income in Wisconsin in 2004 was $19.1 billion, or $11,155 per year per two-income family.

We now add the health care tax to this amount. Our sum total: **$34,103** per year for a family with two working parents.

WAY FORWARD

We desperately need a comprehensive health reform after the 2008 election. Whoever wins the presidential election will simply have to deal with it—just as he (or she) will have to deal with social security. We all agree, one way or the other, that we do not have a well working health system in America today.

The Democrats have a head start in the health care debate. All their major candidates have already pledged allegiance to a single payer system. Their support troops in, e.g., the unions are squarely behind the single payer strategy. Their state parties are working hard to test the waters for single payer systems—to gain more legislative experience in how to handle the issue, and to see how Republicans respond.

If the Republicans want to catch up and present a credible alternative, they better act now. Instead of poking around in little things, like tax breaks that can easily be repealed by a tax-hungry Congress, they should use the Romney model as a platform and enhance it in accordance with the check list I discussed earlier:

- Build a national Connector where insurance plans from all across the country can be sold nationally.

- Create a small business pool that gives them leverage and ERISA exemptions

- Single state registration of insurance plans: any plan registered in one state can be offered nationally through the Connector.

- Delay insurance requirement for individuals—let the free market work prove that it can do its job first.

- Preserve Medicaid for the poor and promote self determination for as many people as possible.

- No price regulations—competition and consumer choice are better at keeping costs down than the government.

This check list addresses all the critical aspects of health reform. The most important aspect is the onerous state-level coverage mandates. The check list does away with them by allowing any registered health plan to be sold nationally. By doing so, it helps Congress comply with the Constitution's Article I, Section 8, Clause 3—a.k.a., the Commerce Clause. State coverage mandates are barriers to interstate commerce, and since it is one of the federal government's core duties to guarantee interstate commerce, it is only logical to challenge state coverage mandates under the Commerce Clause.

Last Congress, the 109th, had the chance to do this. Congressman John Shadegg (R-AZ) proposed a bill, the Health Care Choice Act, that would have neutralized the state mandates. Unfortunately, the Republican majority did not think it was an important enough issue. With a national Romney model it would not be necessary to re-introduce the Shadegg bill. A national insurance "connector" would circumvent the state mandates. States could still keep them—all that matters is that competition is allowed to bring premiums down and consumers get a chance to look for a plan that fits their needs and budgets.

The check list also helps us raise our eyes beyond petty reforms and adherence to group interests that come with tax breaks for employer-based insurance. President Bush has proposed an extension of the health insurance tax credit to cover all private purchases of health insurance, employer-based or not. This is a good idea for the short term: under today's high taxes, many of us will need support from a tax credit to find those last dollars that help us buy insurance.

But tax credits are short lived, especially when their lives are in the hands of a tax hungry Congress. A tax credit is by definition an exception from a norm (the norm being "if it moves, tax it" …) and they also tend to benefit high-income families more than low-income families, simply because high-income families pay more taxes.

That is no reason not to have tax credits, but it would be a dire mistake if leading Republican presidential contenders thought that everything is hunky-dory with health reform just because we have tax breaks and health savings accounts.

It should be a cinch for Republicans to sign on to a Romney model with these modifications. It should also be easy for sensible, moderate Democrats to sign on to this check list.

But there is one aspect of health reform that the Romney model—even in modified version—does not deal with: tort reform.

Fortunately, this is an area where things are already happening. During the '90s Americans in general began to grow tired of ridiculous medical malpractice lawsuits. In the middle of that decennium, studies showed, tort costs on the American economy exceeded $150 billion. That's a lot of cash. It's enough to buy you 150,000 two-bedroom apartments on Manhattan, or one million handsomely equipped Mercedes SL600 ... All that money went to pay for medical lawsuits. Some was undoubtedly warranted, but there were a huge number of cases that were little more than masked extortion.

The damage done by excessive litigation is highly visible in states that have passed meaningful tort reform laws, one of which is Texas. Bill Peacock of the Texas Public Policy Foundation has documented the vast improvements to the health sector in Texas from tort reform.[41] One of the most important improvements will be visible over the longer term. As the burden of ridiculous compensation shrinks—while people who deserve it still get their compensation—it will be more interesting to doctors to invest time and money in treatments that are higher risk but may cure patients where no cure has thus far been seen. With more high risk treatment methods, more patients survive incurable diseases. Gradually, the high risk methods become low risk methods as the medical profession learns to master them. Costs fall and patients benefit, medically as well as financially.

On top of this, tort reform unclogs the court system by flushing out unwarranted lawsuits. The Texas reform has proven this: there has been a significant drop in medical litigation in the state after the reform bill was signed by the governor.

The best way to assure that tort reform does not go into excesses is to let the states compete with each other. If one state goes too far, it will be recognized by others who will find ways to avoid that mistake.

Through this jurisdictional competition, our states exercise a "checks and balances" control in tort reform. If we allow the federal government to assume a monopoly, or a dominant role, in tort reform, we may have to pay a much higher price for any over-reactions or imperfections that result for such reforms.

So far, tort reform has been a success. Texas has shown the way and we expect the state to continue to do so.

Patience and determination

Again: there is *no magic wand* in health policy. Unless we elect Harry Potter for president, we are going to have to accept that it takes time, commitment and patience to reform our health system. If we elect people in 2008 to carry out health reform, we cannot expect wonders within 2–3 years. It will take at least twice as long to see significant results.

Our health system is a behemoth. We spend $2 trillion on health care each year. Such a big industry does not change overnight when we make improvements. Reforms must trickle down and work their way through the system.

As a reminder that time makes a difference, consider this: the reforms that screwed up our system did not, well, screw it up, from one day to the next. It took years before they made health insurance unaffordable for millions of us. By the time that happened, it was difficult at first to see what had really gone wrong.

Obviously, there are many factors behind the high costs of health care. In and by itself, health care is a high-tech product that we cannot buy at Wal-Mart. But precisely for this reason we need to move ahead with the reforms I have sketched here, and summon all our determination as voters/taxpayers/patients to keep the pressure up on our legislators.

There is a lot in the balance. If we do nothing about our health care system, we will only give green light to a destructive status quo. If we do the wrong thing, more people will end up without insurance. Quick fixes like tax breaks or more Medicaid are only cosmetics on a wound that needs comprehensive treatment.

Free market reforms, coupled with determination and patience, will be the best cure to ensure lasting reform going. That combo is perhaps the weakest link in our political chain. Our politicians may be determined, but they are not always very patient. Sometimes it is almost as though patience and political results are mutually exclusive.

But that does not mean that we, the people, should forget to be patient. As they say on the Klingon home world …: Patience is a human virtue. Our patience and our determination to give health reform time and let it deliver, will eventually make the difference between failure and success. If we abandon market-oriented reforms half way, we will end up with an even worse mess than we have now.

In 2008 we have the chance of the century to elect someone who will take the lead in reforming our health system. Let's take that chance.

Endnotes

1. See the Governor's own website: http://mittromney.com/Learn-About-Mitt/Mittxs_Biography.

2. The next chapter explains this figure.

3. See my article, "The Health Care Choice Act: Restoring Competition in the Health Insurance Market", *Prosperitas*, Center for Freedom and Prosperity, June 2006. Available at: http://www.freedomandprosperity.org/Papers/hc-choice/hc-choice.pdf

4. Kip Sullivan: "Massachusetts' 'Universal Coveage' Bill is No Such Thing", *In These Times*, May 7, 2006. Available at: http://www.inthesetimes.com/site/main/article/2639/.

5. Julie Appleby: "Average family policy nears $11,000", *USA Today*, September 14, 2005. Available at: http://www.usatoday.com/money/industries/health/2005-09-14-family-health-policy_x.htm?POE=click-refer.

6. Alice Dembner: "Change in health care law urged", *The Boston Globe and boston.com*, January 25, 2007. Available at: http://www.boston.com/news/local/articles/2007/01/25/change_in_healthcare_law_urged/.

7. There is no such thing as a solution "forever" to any complex social and economic problem. Anyone who tells you otherwise does not know what he is talking about. All we can do is our best to solve problems, like unaffordable insurance, as best we can for as long into the future as possible. What we do know is that government-run entitlement programs come with more long term problems than market based solutions. (Need we say more than Social Security…?) Therefore, the Romney model is a promising alternative, at least at the national level.

8. Bureau of the Census; American Community Survey 2005; Income, Earnings and Poverty. Available at: http://www.census.gov/hhes/www/income/incomestats.html.

9. David L Englin: "Double Duty: Liberals should make the case for universal health care on national-security grounds", *The American Prospect*, January 17, 2003. Available at: http://www.prospect.org/webfeatures/2003/01/englin-d-01-17.html.

10. See my article: "Competition and Consumer Choice—An Option to Universal Health Care in North Carolina"; *Conservative Citizen*; John William Pope Civitas Institute, Winter 2006–2007. Available at: http://www.jwpcivitasinstitute. org/newsroom/Magazine/Winter%2006%20Magazine.pdf.

11. The United States National Health Insurance Act, HR 676, introduced by Represenatives Conyers, Kucinich, McDermott and Christensen. Available at: http://www.house.gov/conyers/news_hr676_2.htm.

12. Michael M Bates: "John Edwards and universal health care", *MichNews.com*, January 3, 2007. Available at: http://www.michnews.com/artman/publish/article_15295.shtml.

13. Glen Johnson: "Kerry Proposes Universal Coverage by 2012", *ABC News Politics*, July 31, 2006. Available at: http://abcnews.go.com/Politics/wireStory?id=2256814&CMP=OTC-RSSFeeds0312.

14. Theoretically, of course, in a socialist country like Cuba everything is not only covered, but everything is "free". In practice, though, there are severe shortages in the Cuban health system—just as in the Soviet system—which of course means that most people do not get nearly all the health care they need.

15. Wesley J Smith: "The English Patient", *The Weekly Standard*, May 30, 2005. Available at: http://www.weeklystandard.com/Content/Public/Articles/000/000/005/645igjun.asp?pg=2.

16. See footnote 10.

17. CESifo DICE: Social Policy Data; Poverty and Income Distribution. Available at: http://www.cesifo. de/pls/diceguest/download/Poverty,%20Income%20Distribution/Gov-benef-tax-subs.pdf.

18. Clifford Kraus: "Canadian high court opens door for sale of health insurance:, *San Francisco Chronicle*, June 10, 2005. Available at: http://www.sfgate.com/cgi-bin/article.cgi?f=/c/a/2005/06/10/MNG8SD6BU11.DTL&type=health.

19. Joe Schneider: "Canadian Court Paves Way for Private Health Insurance", *Bloomberg.com* via Pacific Research Institute, June 9, 2005. Available at: http://www.pacificresearch.org/press/clip/2005/clip-06-09-05.html.

20. Nadeem Esmail, Michael A Walker and Dominika Wrona: "Hospital Waiting Lists in Canada", *Critical Issues Bulletin 2006*, The Fraser Institute, Vancouver, BC. Available at: http://www.fraserinstitute.ca/admin/books/chapterfiles/WYT2006part1.pdf#.

21. Sean Parnell: "Long Waits for Health Care Plague Canada", *Health Care News*, The Heartland Institute, January 1, 2006. Available at: http://www.heartland.org/Article.cfm?artId=18276.

22. Toronto Star, Toronto, Ont., April 22, 2006, Pg. A19.

23. Jeremy Hurst and Luigi Siciliani: "Tackling Excessive Waiting Times for Elective Surgery", *OECD Health Working Papers*, OECD, Paris, France 2003. Available at: http://www.oecd.org/dataoecd/24/32/5162353.pdf.

24. Jeremy Hurst and Luigi Siciliani: "Explaining Waiting-Time Variations for Elective Surgery Across OECD Countries", *OECD Economic Studies*, OECD, Paris, France 2004. Available at: http://www.oecd.org/dataoecd/15/52/35028282.pdf.

25. *Sundsvalls Tidning*, January 21, 2007. Available at: http://st.nu/nyheter/lokalt.php?action=visa_artikel&id=613717.

26. *Aftonbladet*, December 3, 2006. Available at: http://www.aftonbladet.se/vss/nyheter/story/0,2789,945769,00.html.

27. *Aftonbladet*, December 6, 2006. Available at: http://www.aftonbladet.se/vss/nyheter/story/0,2789,948519,00.html.

28. Physicians for National Health Insurance, Mission Statement. Available at: http://www.pnhp.org.

29. *Gavle Dagblad*, various articles. Available at: http://gd.se/Article.jsp?article=57152 and http://gd.se/Article.jsp?article=73150 and http://gd.se/Article.jsp?article=39686.

30. Alfonzo, Schuknecht and Tanzi: "Public Sector Efficiency: An International Comparison", *Working Paper 2003/242*, European Central Bank. Available at: http://www.ecb.int/pub/pdf/scpwps/ecbwp242.pdf.

31. Bureau of the Census: "Income, Poverty and Health Insurance Coverage in the United States 2005", especially Table 8, page 22. *Current Population Reports*. Available at: http://www.census.gov/prod/2006pubs/p60-231.pdf.

32. Not all of them are working, but by dividing the personal income by all of them, we can also divide the health care taxes by all of them. Thereby we get the lowest possible tax burden that we can come up with. In reality, the state of California will have to squeeze more money out of each taxpayer, since only some 80–85 percent of all working age Californians can be expected to actively earn a taxable income.

33. This figure is an estimate based on how much taxes we pay on our personal incomes. Individual families will, of course, pay less or more depending on actual income, deductions and the number of brackets in the income tax code. (This note also applies to the numbers for the individual states.)

34. http://www.cga.ct.gov/2006/TOB/s/pdf/2006SB-00482-R00-SB.pdf.

35. http://www.senatedems.ct.gov/pr/defronzo-060929.html. Italics added.

36. http://cthealth.server101.com/index.html.

37. United Health Care, Network plan. Source: http://ehealthinsurance.com.

38. These numbers are all available at the Bureau of Labor Statistics website. The tables you would want to look for are "State and County Employment and Wages from the Quarterly Census of Employment and Wages", http://www.bls.gov/data/home.htm. Unfortunately, this database only goes back to 2001, but looking at one year alone is revealing enough.

39. http://www.legis.state.wi.us/2005/data/fe/SB-388fe.pdf

40. Department of Administration of the State of Wisconsin, Division of Executive Budget and Finance, Fiscal Estimate for SB 388, 2005 Legislative Session.

41. Bill Peacock: "Restoring Civil Justice in Texas", *Policy Perspective*; Texas Public Policy Foundation, April 2006. Available at: http://www.texaspolicy.com/pdf/2006-04-PP-tortreform-bp.pdf.

978-0-595-43732-
0-595-43732-X